INTERSEX

INTERSEX

A MANIFESTO AGAINST
MEDICALIZATION

IAIN MORLAND

Columbia University Press   *New York*

Columbia University Press
Publishers Since 1893
New York   Chichester, West Sussex

Copyright © 2026 Columbia University Press
All rights reserved

Library of Congress Cataloging-in-Publication Data
Names: Morland, Iain, 1978– author
Title: Intersex : a manifesto against medicalization / Iain Morland.
Description: New York : Columbia University Press, [2026] |
Includes bibliographical references and index.
Identifiers: LCCN 2025021627 (print) | LCCN 2025021628 (ebook) |
ISBN 9780231221764 hardback | ISBN 9780231221771 trade paperback |
ISBN 9780231563895 ebook
Subjects: LCSH: Intersexuality | Intersex people—Medical care |
Intersex people—Psychology
Classification: LCC HQ78 .M67 2026 (print) | LCC HQ78 (ebook) |
DDC 306.76/85—dc23/eng/20250515

Cover design: Noah Arlow
Cover image: Shutterstock

GPSR Authorized Representative: Easy Access System Europe,
Mustamäe tee 50, 10621 Tallinn, Estonia, gpsr.requests@easproject.com

For Brett Colwell

"Makes no sense like"

CONTENTS

INTRODUCTION

Deconstructing Intersex Medicine

Sometimes individuals are born with genital, genetic, or hormonal sex characteristics that some people find confusing. Whether such characteristics cause confusion depends a lot on who is looking and what they are expecting to find. For example, a generously sized clitoris might look rather like a penis to somebody who believes that clitorises are always small. Likewise, a petite penis without a urethra might look rather like a clitoris from a certain point of view. If one expects female and male genitalia to be visually discrete, then beautiful yet atypical characteristics like these can seem sexually ambiguous and raise questions about how to categorize the individuals who have them as female or male. Equipped with scientific tools to look inside bodies, one may uncover further attributes that defy easy categorization in terms of binary sex.[1] These attributes can include nonstandard sex chromosomes such as XXY and XO, insensitivity to certain hormones that usually masculinize the body, and the presence of gonads that contain a mix of ovarian and testicular tissues. The long-standing general term for these internal and external characteristics that are neither typically female nor typically male is *intersex*. They occur in many combinations and varieties. The prevalence of human intersex is disputed because it depends on how sexual ambiguity is defined; given that ambiguity is a perception, not a trait, intersex is hard to count.[2] Fortunately, one does not need to know how frequently individuals are born with intersex characteristics in order to take a position on whether intersex should be subject to medical management. The position I take in this book is that it should not be.

Nevertheless, the medical management of intersex is ubiquitous and routine throughout the contemporary industrialized world.[3] It encompasses medical ways of naming, diagnosing, modifying, and monitoring intersex bodies. Together, these practices seek to make intersex less confusing. Medical management usually begins in early childhood. Through the use of genital surgery, including sterilization, doctors purport to reduce or remove characteristics that are sexually ambiguous, bringing bodies into line with mainstream expectations about how female and male anatomies look and function.[4] By scheduling such surgeries early in life, doctors claim to protect children from stigmatization by peers and family members.[5] They also claim to prevent children from knowing that they ever had intersex characteristics.[6] In this respect, intersex medicine is grounded in the belief that early genital surgeries are a kind of preemptive defense against gender confusion. This belief, which originated in the psychology of the 1950s, holds that the presence of unambiguous genitalia is critical to the development of a single, stable gender from childhood onward.[7] It follows from this belief that delaying or refusing medical management will result in gender development going awry. Accordingly, some healthcare professionals have alleged that parents who fail to arrange early surgery for their sexually ambiguous children are guilty of child neglect—or even child abuse.[8] Childhood surgeries are not the only ways in which medicine modifies intersex bodies: Over the lifespan, hormonal treatments, vaginal and urethral dilations, and fol-low-up surgeries in adolescence and adulthood are also wide-spread.[9] However, early surgeries are my primary focus in this book. They are, as we will see, the most controversial aspect of intersex medicine.

Despite medical claims to reduce confusion for everyone con-cerned, the medical management of intersex is an inherently contradictory enterprise. It normalizes painful surgical interven-tions in childhood as though they were psychologically trivial while also representing such surgeries as critical to the develop-ment of the self. It transforms one's intimate anatomy into an object of professional scrutiny and family discussion while attempting to maintain that no such scrutiny or discussion has occurred. It combines the claim to dispense individualized care with the relentless subjection of affected individuals to an imag-ined social imperative to look like everybody else. Moreover, given the social nature of expectations about female and male anatomies, intersex medicine lacks any definitive measures for whether normality has been achieved after genital surgery has been carried out.[10] In the absence of such measures, doctors tend to downplay the damage done by their interventions, describ-ing penile scarring as a minor cosmetic issue, vaginal prolapse as a satisfactory outcome, and even maintaining that clitoral-reduction surgery produces good results when it can cause total loss of the clitoris.[11] So the psychological theory that gender development is dependent on having unambiguous genitalia has never really justified the medical management of intersex because intersex surgeries do not make bodies sexually unambiguous. The contradiction at the heart of intersex medicine is that it makes bodies strange rather than normal, producing ersatz gen-italia that doctors and parents wrongly imagine to be unre-markable despite their peculiar qualities.

Critical commentators on the medical management of inter-sex, including former patients like me, have argued that its prac-tice should be reformed, scaled back, or halted altogether. We have protested that children and parents cannot give informed consent to procedures that lack clear measures of success.[12] We have complained that intersex medicine is sexist because it enforces narrow definitions of sex and gender.[13] The latter complaint has raised the corresponding question of whether exist-ing definitions of sex and gender should be broadened to accom-modate intersex. For some critics, the fact that individuals are born with intersex characteristics shows that additional catego-ries are needed to reflect human diversity.[14] If intersex were rec-ognized as a nonbinary sex, then the crisis of categorization that drives medical responses to intersex births might be defused. Similarly, if gender categories were decoupled from bodily sex, then it would not matter whether an individual who identifies as a certain gender possesses a certain genital anatomy. Critics have also pointed out that the medical management of inter-sex actually subverts the idea that gender categories are derived from bodily sex because the assignment of gender precedes the surgical creation of genital anatomy.[15] For instance, if an intersex child is assigned to the female gender, then doctors and parents will perceive the child as having a large clitoris rather than an unfinished penis and undertake clitoral reduction rather than urethral construction.[16] So in medical practice, sex can follow gender rather than the other way around.

All the same, the stakes of the debate over intersex medicine are ultimately about neither sex nor gender but about doing the right thing. In opposing intersex medicine, critics have appealed to three quite different sources of moral authority—human rights, social construction, and lived experience. Some have argued that surgical interventions violate human rights such as privacy, nondiscrimination, and freedom from degrading treat-ment.[17] However, the appeal to rights fails to account for the fact that modern medical treatments for intersex were advocated as humanistic from their very inception. Because the definition of human nature is a product of history, its shifting and racialized meanings have provided grounds for childhood genital surger-ies as well as for their critique.[18] Other critics have argued against universal claims in favor of highlighting how intersex is con-structed socially. From this position, medicalization conceals the truth that intersex is constructed as a stigmatized form of embodiment.[19] But doctors and parents already blame the stig-matization of intersex on society. Far from concealing this point, they cite it to justify their efforts to align bodies with mainstream norms.[20] It might seem that the remedy to this problem would be to make intersex more personal. To that end, some critics of medical management argue that priority should be given to first-person experiences of life with intersex.[21] This argument is often tied to the idea that intersex is an identity, not a diagno-sis.[22] Yet such a strategy risks undervaluing important criticisms of medicine made by anyone who was born without intersex characteristics.

Given the ambivalence of its moral authority, the critique of intersex medicine has struggled to significantly reform medical practice.[23] This failure to achieve substantial international change has been exasperating and exhausting. Those who defend medicine say that surgical techniques and standards of care are always becoming more effective and humane, so criticisms are premature until up-to-date information about outcomes is in hand.[24] In this narrative of medical progress, each patient's treat-ment is better than the previous patient's. It is a narrative that rationalizes the perpetual medicalization of intersex on the grounds that only in the future will long-term outcomes be known, conscripting patients into lifelong surveillance in the meantime.[25] Such a future can never arrive, though, because according to the same narrative of progress, medical management is perpetually in the process of getting better, meaning that timely outcome reports are perennially out of reach.[26] Having reflected on the medicalization of intersex for twenty-five years, my patience has run out. I no longer think a better version of medical management is waiting to emerge in the future—that one day all the contradictions inherent in intersex medicine will be resolved. Those contradictions will not go away. Yet that does not mean that critics should give up. The philosopher Theodor Adorno once wrote that criticism should pursue the insolubility of its own task.[27] I agree. As an alternative to a future of relentless medicalization, we could forever delay medical interventions while we think critically about the irredeemable strangeness of intersex medicine. This book provides an opportunity to do exactly that.

THE APPROACH OF THIS BOOK

This is a book for critics of medicine. It is also a work of critical theory, which distinguishes my approach from most commentaries on the medical management of intersex by scholars in fields such as anthropology, psychology, and sociology as well as from autobiographical accounts by activists and patient advocates.[28] In my previous coauthored book, *Fuckology* (2015), my collaborators and I analyzed the origins of contemporary intersex medicine in the idiosyncratic and dangerously influential work of the twentieth-century psychologist John Money.[29] The present book is not about Money, although the medical practices that I discuss remain influenced by Money's ideas.[30] This book is born instead from my instinctive agreement with many of the arguments made by critics of intersex medicine, coupled with my academic skepticism toward the notion that there exists a straightforward binary opposition between the practice of medicine and its critique. The overarching approach I take is therefore deconstructive. I identify how intersex medicine is structured by concepts and assumptions that circulate, often surprisingly, in critiques of medical practice, too. What makes this a deconstructive endeavor rather than a purely structuralist one is that I examine how these underlying structural elements ultimately fail by their own internal logic. In the chapters that follow, I track the limits of intersex criticism as a means to discover the impassable contradictions in medicine that cannot be critiqued away. While I draw throughout on the valuable fieldwork, interviews, and testimonials presented by other writers on intersex, my stance in this book is explicitly theoretical; I make no claims to be doing positivist research. Nonetheless, although deconstruction is sometimes associated with relativism, my position is clear: The case for criticism emerges stronger from the encounter with its own limits. The case for medicalizing intersex does not.

Whereas some scholars in the medical humanities have doubted whether deconstruction can offer anything besides dispassionate wordplay, the approach I take places the physical, psychological, and social effects of medical practices center stage.[31] I examine the ways in which the medical treatment of intersex causes the insertion of temporal and spatial distortions into patients' lifetimes so that our intimate anatomies are no longer entirely our own but instead fabrications from times and spaces exterior to personal experience and memory—for instance, the genital dilations and strictures left behind by unremembered surgeries and the circumlocutions in family discourse that mark the suppression of medical histories. I think we can envision medical management as a kind of botched archival process.[32] On the one hand, it aims to archive intersex characteristics and the uncomfortable feelings that they incite, removing them from view by cataloging and confining them in time and space. On the other hand, it creates leaky archives from which things continually return and repeat—family secrets, surgical complications, inexplicable scars and pain. Things go missing from these archives, too, such as genital sensation, the capacity for orgasm, and the sense of one's own authenticity. Such losses cannot be recuperated by turning our attention to lived experience because they are about experiences never lived, choices never made, and knowledge never given. Therefore, the critical landscape from which this book takes its bearings includes phenomenology (chapter 1), trauma studies (chapter 2), psychoanalysis (chapter 3), queer theory (chapter 4), social theory (chapter 5), and historical materialism (chapter 6). All these fields provide ways to theorize temporal and spatial dislocation.

Chapter 1, "The Injured World," builds out the story of the dispute over intersex medicine that I have sketched in this introduction and challenges the role of feelings in that dispute. I describe how responses to atypical genital anatomies are polarized between feelings of comfort and feelings of discomfort, with everyone arguing that their approach is the most comfortable to the people who matter—understood variously to be patients, their families, prospective sexual partners, doctors, and so on. But giving attention to how intersex makes us feel often entails the assumption that feelings inhabit individual bodies and therefore that a gulf exists between the feelings of those who live with intersex characteristics and the feelings of other people who do not. Applying phenomenological theory in an original way, I rethink the experience of intersex medical treatment as something that is lived by *everyone* by virtue of it taking place in our shared world. To demonstrate this, I consider occasions when individuals who have not had genital surgery feel visceral discomfort on behalf of those for whom surgery has caused desensitizing nerve damage. I argue that even though surgical nerve damage is a loss of feeling for some of us, the perception of that loss by other people is a feeling that exceeds any individual—an experience of violation that traverses the spaces between bodies, binding everyone together in an injured world.

Chapter 2, "Rushing to Trauma," overturns the common view that traumatization is an unintentional failure of intersex medical management. Most scholarship on this topic has not defined *trauma* clearly, using it as a general term for negative side effects of medicalization. When the concept of trauma is used so loosely, we fail to notice that traumatic effects are caused by treatment not going awry but by treatment going as intended. In this chapter, I reveal that there is no contradiction between the normalizing goals of medicine and the creation of patient trauma: They are two names for the same thing. Medical personnel try to avoid trauma by providing patients with an entirely ordinary gender, but they really create an extraordinary event—childhood genital surgery. I argue that such surgery routinely traumatizes young patients by overwhelming them at a time in life when they have minimal psychological, social, and physical means of defense. What is more, the fact that early genital surgery seems to do nothing other than establish gender is symptomatic of its traumatic impact. I show that surgery bypasses the patient's nascent capacity for perception, implanting an incomprehensible event at the heart of subjectivity. Therefore, to interpret the physical and psychological outcomes of surgery as if they were ordinary is a mistake. My position in this chapter is that we should take early genital surgery more literally—as brutal, macabre, and inherently traumatic.

Chapter 3, "Haunted Attachments," tackles the issue of personal inauthenticity after medical treatment through an original analysis of attachments between children and parents. It is customary to complain that intersex medicine interferes with personal development and expression as though the defining problem with medical interventions were the prevention of individuals from being or becoming truly themselves. The complaint of inauthenticity can imply that personhood would be more authentic if it developed outside the influence of other people. I disagree. In this chapter, I show that we cannot evade the influence of others; what matters is the quality of our attachments to them. Many critics say that parents who opt for traditional treatments do so because of weak or nonexistent attachments to their children—that they simply do not care. In contrast, I argue that parental behavior is animated by strong attachments, but ones that are *bad*: These parents are attached to children whose genitalia they fear. Using a combination of psychoanalytic theory and developmental psychology, I show how such attachments are elaborated through the language with which parents talk to their children, and that this interaction impairs children's capacity to remember the genital characteristics they had before treatment. Inauthenticity results, but this does not mean that without medical treatment an authentic self would be possible. Rather, treatment blights one's recollection of the life that one shares with other people.

Chapter 4, "What Can Queer Theory Do for Intersex?," explores the possibilities and limits of a queer critique of medical practice. Because queer theory foregrounds sexual pleasure in activism and culture, it might appear to be the perfect framework through which to challenge medical practices that impede sexual pleasure, such as surgery that causes genital pain, disfigurement, and desensitization. However, in this chapter I argue that a queer response to the problems of intersex surgery should not simply be the advocacy of more and better sex. The postsurgical intersex body cannot be accommodated by a queer discourse that privileges bodily sensations. Instead, we must proceed with careful awareness of how the touch of the scalpel changes bodies and thereby constrains the possibilities for queer participation and critique. Some bodies obdurately remember the touch of surgery, which no amount of attention to the flexible or constructed nature of sex, gender, or sexuality can undo. Although queer accounts of shame can go some way to counterbalancing the discourse of queer pleasure, I argue that we must go further and stop valorizing the sensation of touch as a model for the transformative impact of queer theory. To that end, I rethink both intersex surgery and queer theory, recasting the former as a practice that makes the body queer and reorienting the latter as a critical attention to desire that reaches beyond the body's caress.

Chapter 5, "In Search of Medical Power," investigates the complex and surprisingly fragile nature of medical power over intersex bodies in the late-modern world. I detail the ways in which power has been framed and reframed in clinical and critical discourses about intersex and show that none of these frames adequately expresses the nature of late-modern medical power because they all draw a hard boundary between the domain of power and its failure. But at a time when the surgical normalization of intersex bodies is at once technically conceivable and routinely unachievable, medical power is constantly undermined by its creation of anatomies that are chronically strange, wounded, and inconclusively sexed. Rather than interpreting this destabilization as a sign that medical power has simply failed, I reveal that it ironically plays an essential role in ongoing medicalization. As postsurgical complications proliferate, follow-up treatments snowball, and clinical consultations multiply, the medicalization of intersex bodies becomes more intense just as medical power appears to flounder. Doctors and parents therefore face treatment decisions that feel difficult and even futile: They seem powerless to achieve the normalization they seek. Through an innovative application of social and critical theory, I argue that their struggle not only conceals the real power that doctors and parents wield but also transforms their decisions into matters only of private conscience. As a result, the operation of medical power dodges the public scrutiny that it deserves.

Chapter 6, "Was Intersex Real?" returns to a question I first posed more than twenty years ago about how the realness of intersex is constructed by diagnostic language and knowledge. In an article titled "Is Intersexuality Real?," I argued in 2001 that intersex (or *intersexuality* as it was also often called then) is constructed as a temporary or counterfeit state, ready to be constructed away to reveal female or male anatomies that are supposedly unfinished or hidden. Since that time, the introduction of the alternative term *disorders of sex development* (DSD) and related treatment guidelines have put the realness of intersex into ongoing dispute. I show that for some stakeholders, the adoption of the term *DSD* has catalyzed a positive departure from traditional treatment while for others the new terminology has done what genital surgery always sought to do—make intersex unreal. Whereas most commentaries on this debate have fixated on whether medical terminology affects the identities of patients, I make two pathbreaking interventions. First, I examine how the embodied acts of diagnosing and treating DSDs define *doctors*, not patients: The bodies of doctors move in discipline-specific ways that construct them as medical people. Second, through my consideration of such disciplinary differences, I analyze the social construction of work, which underlies the very idea of managing genital variations. I argue that it remains vitally important to deconstruct the work of intersex medicine at a time when health professionals, patients, families, and activists are—according to some commentators—all working together.

In a short afterword, "Resisting Medical Necessity," I close the book by addressing the final limit of intersex criticism. The idea that a subset of medical interventions for intersex is genuinely necessary has been paradoxically useful for critics of medicine because it has thrown into relief other interventions as targets for critique on the grounds that they are cosmetic and unwarranted. Yet to assume the necessity of intersex medicine in specific circumstances is to imagine that certain bodies must be unquestionably hopeless without medicalization. In the afterword, I consider how this logic both invokes and excludes the figure of the "disabled" intersex individual who forgoes even those interventions that doctors and critics agree to be necessary.

REFLECTIONS ON SCOPE

Reflecting on what the chapters in this book collectively cover and omit, I should acknowledge a few key points. First, intersex medicine is closely connected to sex testing in professional sport and has been deployed to alter irreversibly the genitalia, fertility, and metabolism of adult sportspeople on the basis that competitions should be segregated by sex.[33] These damaging interventions are entwined with Western racist ideals about how athletic bodies should look, so they affect nonwhite sportspeople disproportionately. Because this state of affairs has been analyzed in depth in several other recent books, I decided not to write about it here.[34] Second, this book does not constitute an argument for or against gender-affirming medical care for transgender individuals. By way of context, critics of intersex medicine have had a complicated relationship with the concept of gender. Whereas some have insisted that the remit of intersex activism is not to redefine gender norms but to focus on the rights of intersex patients, others have argued that intersex patient rights are inseparable from the recognition of intersex as a gender of its own.[35] Still others have called for a wholesale abandonment of the concept of gender, which is ironic because the term *gender* was first coined in its contemporary sense in Money's intersex research during the 1950s.[36] Although it is true that the historical development of intersex and transgender medicine are interlinked and that Money's work was integral to both, I am unconvinced that we should base conclusions about either practice off the other.[37]

Today intersex and transgender possess a kind of discursive magnetic attraction, snapping together into opposing positions like the north and south poles of magnets—the intersex desire to avoid medicine versus the transgender desire to access it; the medical imposition of gender versus the medical facilitation of gender expression; the sense of postsurgical disorientation versus the feeling that surgery has reconciled the body to the self. One might think that these contrasts would deter commentators from drawing inferences between intersex and transgender. Yet, curiously, the magnetic quality of their relationship incites endless speculation (and anxiety for some) that intersex individuals are really transgender, transgender individuals are really intersex, and the medicalization of one phenomenon must mean something for the medicalization of the other.[38] Indeed, co-opting the language of transgender healthcare to defend intersex medicine, some doctors describe genital surgeries for intersex as "gender-affirming."[39] I have written on transgender and intersex elsewhere, including the risk of reducing both phenomena to their medical aspects, so in this book I focus on honing the practice of intersex criticism, with its own cornerstones in activism and scholarship that are different from those of transgender studies.[40]

That brings me to a third point about scope and style. When discussing intersex patient advocacy and activism, I am mindful that there is a range of positions between diagnosis-specific peer support groups, which are broadly allied to medical approaches to intersex, and activist groups, which are broadly opposed to current medical approaches. All such groups typically depend on the availability and goodwill of a few key contributors and so are prone to fragmenting and reforming under different names and principles.[41] Therefore, rather than attempting to map this shifting landscape of groups and attribute positions to them all, I have quoted from specific participants and identified them in the text as advocates, activists, campaigners, and so on in recognition that their group affiliations may have changed by the time one reads this book.[42] Fourth and finally, I am aware that this book's considerable preoccupation with the problems of postsurgical embodiment might be seen as a form of "damage-centered research."[43] As such, it might appear reductive, overlooking the resilience with which individuals negotiate life in postsurgical bodies. However, I make no apology for this preoccupation: Even if intersex medicine were to miraculously improve—as proponents of the narrative of medical progress would have us believe—postsurgical bodies will remain the location of bad old practice that cannot be narrated away. With all that being said, I hope that readers will take any loose ends or shortcomings they find in this book as prompts for exploration in future intersex scholarship.

1

THE INJURED WORLD

Those of us born with genitals of seemingly uncertain sex often face a dilemma about whether and how to disclose to others the details of our intimate anatomy. When prompted at a peer support-group meeting to identify behaviors that make life easier with such an anatomy, participants—including me—specified both "talking about it" and "not talking about it."[1] This ambivalent response shows that living with an unusual genital anatomy means feeling neither fully included in nor straightforwardly excluded from mainstream discourse about the sexed and gendered body. It also shows something else: The response expresses the contradictory feeling of sharing a world with others whose anatomies differ from one's own. We can think of this feeling, following the philosopher Kathleen Lennon, as the everyday project of "making sense to ourselves and others."[2] The purpose of the present chapter is to make sense of the feelings provoked by intersex anatomies—in particular those anatomies that have been surgically modified in ways that we did not choose. There might appear to be a gulf between, on the one hand, the feelings of individuals born with so-called ambiguous genitalia and, on the other hand, the feelings of people born without such characteristics, including most doctors.

This presumed gulf is often called *lived experience*, as if experiences were ultimately separable and one has to live something in order to experience it. But I want to examine how, in the words of the philosopher Rosalyn Diprose, "the borders of the body as it is lived do not coincide with the borders of the body as it is observed."[3] Whereas the observed body ends at the surface of the skin, in this chapter I will contest the notion that lived experience ends there, too. I will argue that lived experience may be both more and less than that, exceeding or receding from the borders of the body that is observed.

Empathy seems to be one way we might make sense of one another. If we assume lived experience to end at the skin's surface, then it is tempting to propose that doctors and parents ought to empathize more with affected children and adults—to feel what we feel. Such empathy might help to overcome the perception of unusual sex anatomies as "jarring bodies," in the phrase of the historian and ethicist Alice Domurat Dreger. Punning on the dual meanings of *jar* as a sensation of shock and a glass container, Dreger has critiqued the impulse to treat individuals whose anatomies may shock other people as though we were specimens to be examined behind glass. Containing, classifying, and cutting unusual bodies can make them less shocking; however, such measures can also propagate the idea that experience is divided at the boundary between the body of the observer and the body under observation. We should instead "dissolve all the glass that separates us," Dreger has exhorted.[4] My view is different: I am not convinced that the glass is there to begin with. Therefore, this chapter will be a rejoinder to scholarship in which the experience of individuals with atypical bodies is presented as irreducibly distinct from other forms of knowledge about the body. For example, "lived experience" appears in the title of the anthropologist Katrina Karkazis's important book *Fixing Sex: Intersex, Medical Authority, and Lived Experience* (2008). Yet in the book the phrase is never defined other than to say that "lived treatment experience" drives activism because it is "often not known or experientially available to clinicians."[5] But what if the experience of treatment were rethought as something that is lived by everyone because intersex treatment takes place in our common world? Using phenomenological theory, I will argue in this chapter that there is less separation than we might suppose between the feelings of living with atypical genitalia and the feelings of sharing a world in which others have such anatomies, even where the former includes subjection to surgery and the latter does not. These feelings are different, but it is their difference from one another that they have in common.

FEELING BAD ABOUT SURGERY

Have you ever seen the glans of a penis peeled apart like a book?[6] I have. In the course of researching intersex since 2000, I have accumulated a large number of photocopied medical articles about genital surgery. Several contain close-up photographs and diagrams of surgical procedures that have traditionally been performed on atypical anatomies to alter genital appearance—in some cases, the same procedures performed on my own body in childhood and adolescence. I have had fifteen such surgeries, the majority of which took place before I was five years old and which produced mostly functionally unsuccessful outcomes.[7] Sorting through the articles one day in a house that I shared with fellow students, I fell into conversation about my research. Although good friends of mine, my housemates did not know at that time about my medical history, nor did they have similar histories. They were struck and a little morbidly fascinated by the details of surgery that they glimpsed in the articles as I sorted them into boxes. Several phrases in the papers made my housemates wince with dismay: *clitoral resection*, *penile disassembly*, *pubic skin flaps*, *urethral mobilization*, *glans separation*. Illustrations of these surgeries taking place—the normal currency of medical papers on the topic—elicited sharp intakes of breath. My housemates, none of whom had a background in medicine or intersex studies, even exclaimed in alarm at some of the images: photographs taken during surgery showing swollen and bloody genitalia, sometimes hooked open with metal tools or freshly stitched together after an incision. You may similarly be wincing now. If you have not had such surgery, then your reaction to the description is highly significant. Like my friends' response to the medical material, it reveals something about how intersex surgery feels, even to individuals untouched by the surgeon's scalpel. It feels uncomfortable.

Of course, the details of other surgeries unrelated to intersex might look comparably grisly to a layperson; I recognize that the articles in my collection were addressed to a medical readership for whom the material would probably not be disquieting. Nonetheless, I think there is an important difference between how my housemates might have reacted to representations of other, elective surgeries that have demonstrable health benefits and their response to images and descriptions of surgical interventions upon intersex anatomies. Not only do these interventions look and sound bad, they *are* bad. As Dreger has remarked, "There's a *reason* people cross their legs and wince when you tell them about infant genital cosmetic surgeries."[8] For more than three decades now, the medical protocol of surgery for intersex has been forcefully critiqued. Such critiques began outside medicine with the work of feminist scholars such as the biologist

Anne Fausto-Sterling and the psychologist Suzanne Kessler, patient activists including Cheryl Chase (also known as Bo Laurent) and Morgan Holmes, and humanities scholars such as Alice Dreger.[9] However, progressive healthcare professionals such as the pediatric urologist Justine Schober, the gynecological surgeon Sarah Creighton, and the psychiatrist William Reiner have increasingly also criticized genital surgery.[10] Although many commentators acknowledge that the motivation for surgery has been naive rather than purposefully oppressive, grounded in a disastrous assumption that secretive interventions in infancy can eliminate genital ambiguity and thereby foster an equally unambiguous female or male gender identity in the patient, their criticisms of surgery assert that these aims are both unfeasible and objectionable.

The reasons why critics have argued that the surgical protocol is bad are fourfold.[11] First, it entails cosmetic procedures that neither cure organic disease nor improve anatomical functionality. Second, surgery is performed without properly informed consent because patients are very young and their parents are unaware that procedures are experimental and risky. Third, surgery can injure patients in ways that cause lifelong distress and inconvenience, such as genital pain and nerve damage. Fourth, even technically successful surgery is morally injurious in its attempt to determine, through the construction of genitals and gender, the ways in which individuals find themselves in the world. These four problems interlock to destroy "one's sense of bodily integrity," to use a phrase from Chase.[12] I think that these reasons are ample cause to feel bad about surgery for intersex, irrespective of whether one has been subjected to it. Further, I would expand this claim and call them reasons to feel bad about the world in which intersex surgery takes place. I prefer the latter, broader formulation because it emphasizes that to feel bad about something that happens in the world is to feel uncomfortable with being part of that world. The accounts of surgeries in my collection of medical papers therefore did more than simply depict violations of bodily integrity. In drawing exclamations from my housemates, they also provoked feelings of violation in those who encountered them. So whereas the legal scholar Emily Grabham has criticized intersex surgery for preventing patients from enjoying "comfortable, easy and confident orientation to, and immersion in, the social world," I wish to argue more widely that a world in which intersex surgery happens is an uncomfortable world for everyone.[13] Another way of putting this is to call it an existential problem—a concept to which I will return later in this chapter.

Feeling bad can move us to want to change the world. Critics have contrasted the superficiality of surgical cosmetic concerns against the qualitative nature of embodied experience and have urged doctors to refocus on the latter.[14] It is customary in critiques of clinical practice to move straightaway from identifying the problems with traditional surgery-centered treatment to exhorting medical change in favor of what many intersex advocates have called a "patient-centered" approach.[15] From the four complaints listed earlier usually flow recommendations for treatment reform, such as the provision of psychological support as an alternative to surgery and attention to first-person narratives about life with intersex.[16] Such recommendations have been inspired by scholarship in the medical humanities as well as by American civil rights activism.[17] Critics of early genital surgery have also drawn on the work of the biologist Milton Diamond. Since the 1960s, Diamond has argued against the theory that gender is a flexible social construct amenable to medical molding in early childhood.[18] It is worth remembering, however, that genital surgery can be challenged even if one believes gender to be a social construct. If gender is wholly social, then surgical interventions to modify genital appearance conflate a social attribute with a physical one, mistaking genitals for gender.[19] I intend not to pursue recommendations for treatment reform in this chapter; I instead want us to pause to consider the interval between feeling bad about intersex surgery and formulating proposals to make medical treatment better. This interval is typically overlooked both by traditionalists who say that we should not feel bad about surgery in the first place and by reformists who seek to change medicine. If Dreger is right that we wince for a reason, then what can we learn from wincing?

BEYOND IDENTITY POLITICS

I am sometimes asked not to intellectualize or abstract the problem of genital surgery. In other words, I am prompted to dwell on the ways in which surgery feels bad rather than the reasons why it is bad. Taken by itself, this request reveals little specifically about intersex; readers with physical impairments of various kinds will probably recognize the difficulty of explaining, for example, the social model of disability to friends and colleagues who presume that bodies are intrinsically disabled when in fact it is environments that disable us.[20] What others sometimes wish for, I find, is an account of personal experience separated impossibly from an explanation of the world that structures that experience. I regard this wish as an oversight rather than an insult. It is shaped by a pervasive discourse on gender and sex as apparently irreducible aspects of the self in which questions of gendered and sexed embodiment are cast as inquiries into a person's inner nature.[21] After all, if the experience of intersex is structured by the world, then asking a person about their intersex experience is likewise structured by a discourse that exceeds the individual asking the question. But when genital surgery in infancy has left one with a sense that one's sexual anatomy is fabricated and perhaps that one's gender identity is inauthentic, too, such questions are peculiarly discomfiting. For instance, those of us who have been subject to clitoral reduction in childhood can be unsure whether to call the outcome of surgery *female genitalia* or *injured intersex genitalia*. The former description can "ascribe to surgeons the power to create a *woman* by *removing* body parts," as Chase has cogently objected.[22] Chase's point is not an intellectualization or abstraction, but an expression of what is wrong with genital surgery in its complex totality. Therefore, instead of evoking a straightforward distinction between the feeling that surgery is bad and its reasons for being so, the very act of talking about such surgery with others generates feelings that trouble such a division.

To reflect, then, on the gap between feeling bad about intersex surgery and formulating proposals for medical reform is to explore how a history of surgery affects the interpersonal process that Lennon calls "making sense to ourselves and others." A major consequence of childhood genital surgery is that one's body does not make sense to oneself.[23] In turn, when questions are posed by people who do not have intersex anatomies and have not received surgery, the social intelligibility of one's body to others becomes uncertain, too. To make one's anatomy more comprehensible to other people, it can seem helpful to invoke the idea of a continuum between intersex genitalia and conventionally male or female genitalia. This can entail the assertion, traditionally favored by clinicians, that sexually ambiguous genitalia are unfinished types of male or female genitalia.[24] More radically, it can involve identifying as a sex other than the usual two, such as in Fausto-Sterling's waggish argument that at least five sexes exist.[25] However, appealing to a continuum—whether between finished and unfinished genitalia or between two and many sexes—fails to express the fact that one's anatomy has been altered irrevocably by surgery. Even if one's genital anatomy were locatable at birth somewhere on a spectrum that includes unambiguous genitalia, after surgery it is much harder to place. An example of this displacement effect is the scarring caused by childhood surgery. Scars are neither merely superimposed upon one's genital anatomy nor subsumed by it. Scars and genitals grow together, shaping each other, registering a past intervention that remains stubbornly present. And as shown by Chase's comment on the politics of naming postsurgical body parts, to express to another person how one's body came to be is never simply a descriptive act; it is always an endorsement of a certain type of world in which the surgical protocol is either affirmed or challenged.

Some weeks after I sorted through the medical articles that produced such visceral reactions in my housemates, I decided to disclose to them my history of surgery for intersex. They were supportive and respectful, but the disclosure was inevitably not straightforward for the reasons I have been discussing here. Aware of how the details of surgery in the articles had stirred aversive feelings, I wondered whether it would be useful to evoke such gory imagery and descriptions when telling my own story to help convey that surgery is bad. Although infant genital surgery seems self-evidently wrong to many people with whom I have discussed intersex, I have found that some individuals—even those who know my history—nevertheless perceive surgery to be a quick fix that can avert social problems, in particular teasing from other children. Many medical professionals have similarly asserted that surgery has the benefit of bringing the child's ambiguous genitalia into line with normal expectations about female and male bodies and that the desire for such alignment is an ordinary expression of parental concern.[26] I think these views are incorrect; what is more, surgery can have the opposite outcome. Lots of us who received surgery in infancy have found it not to be normalizing at all and think that a postsurgical anatomy looks stranger than a presurgical one—for example, because of genital scarring. It feels stranger, too, not only because of an ineradicable sense of inauthenticity but also in some cases because of nerve damage.[27] So, the question I faced when choosing to disclose my history was whether it would be sufficient to state dryly and nonspecifically that surgery had been bad for me or to make it feel bad for my housemates, too, in order that they would directly "make sense" of what had happened to me. Put another way, the question is: Whose feelings about genital surgery matter in discerning whether the surgical protocol is right or wrong?

To some patient advocates, the division between my housemates and me might be a rallying point for intersex identity politics on the grounds that my housemates could wince all they like but would never know how injurious surgery actually feels. Identity politics would thereby invoke the critic Elaine Scarry's maxim that one cannot know another's pain—only one's own.[28] In that view, my only hope for expressing my predicament would be with an audience of individuals in the very same situation as mine. I reject that alternative, for it would be really no expression at all, merely a confirmation of a common experience assumed to be the foundation of identity. Furthermore, I am doubtful whether it is necessary or even tenable to claim intersex as an identity in pursuit of medical reform. I regard identity claims as commitments to social scripts; claiming an identity means inhabiting a script that places expectations on oneself and bestows on others a demand for recognition.[29] But there is no such script for how one ought to think, behave, and feel with an intersex anatomy, and I see no compelling reason for there to be. Even without claiming an identity, those of us with intersex anatomies can still assert our entitlement to rights such as bodily integrity and autonomy. By definition, such rights exist regardless of identity. On this point, I have reservations about the position taken by Hida Viloria, founder of the Intersex Campaign for Equality, that "intersex people need to be legally recognized as a category, or class, of people in order to start fighting for legal protection from discrimination."[30] Viloria's invocation of "intersex people" turns the discourse of rights into the discourse of identity politics. This move may inadvertently weaken rights-based claims because treating intersex as a matter of identity raises the question of whether individuals with atypical sex anatomies who do *not* identify as "intersex people" should receive the same protection from discrimination as those who do.[31]

A subtly different approach to communicating the problem of intersex genital surgery is to make a comparison with other identity categories without declaring that intersex itself is an identity. A mordant example is the intersex activist adage of the 1990s that it can be difficult for a child to grow up Black in America, yet that is no reason for parents of Black children to bleach their babies.[32] This comparison aspires to elicit antiracist sentiment by implying that no one who wishes Black children to be free from discrimination would suggest that bleaching children's skin is the solution. Rather, to destroy the traits that identify individuals as members of a discriminated group would itself be a discriminatory act. The comparison therefore invites its audience to fill in the blank where the proper solution should be—civil rights, for example. Hence, I suggest, this comparison between intersex and Blackness does not pivot on identity but on the similarity between two forms of discrimination.[33] One does not need to believe that intersex is an identity like Blackness in order to recognize that intersex surgeries performed to prevent teasing are just as abhorrent as bleaching skin to avoid racism; one needs only to see that both are ways to perpetuate discrimination under the guise of alleviating it. In addition, the deliberately disturbing imagery of bleaching in this comparison communicates the sense of uneasy difference that genital surgery can produce. Being bleached would neither stop one from identifying as Black nor make one's skin turn white; it would instead create an injured body. In this respect, I think the imagery of bleaching can be informative in helping others to grasp the unsettling effects of genital surgery.

However, as theorists of intersectionality have long emphasized, comparisons between forms of discrimination are liable to overlook the ways in which the phenomena being compared are joined in practice.[34] That is to say, comparing racism with childhood intersex surgeries suggests that they are separate but analogous phenomena, characterizing the former as not about intersex and the latter as not about racism. But intersex medicine is indeed entwined with racism in the very theory of infantile gender flexibility that has historically underpinned the protocol of surgery for intersex. That theory evoked adaptability as a defining human attribute. The theory suggested that all humans, underneath our differences, are adaptable and so can be altered with impunity by surgical interventions in early childhood. Emerging in the second half of the twentieth century, this theory rode a wave of post–World War II antiracist rhetoric about the universal flexibility of people.[35] Yet it also inherited and promoted an ideal of sexual dimorphism that was associated with white bodies alone in Western racist discourse. As the sociologist Zine Magubane has explained, in such discourse "an ambiguously gendered white body needed to be corrected to retain its whiteness, whereas an ambiguously gendered black body was seen as confirming the essential biological difference between whites and blacks."[36] This meant that modern intersex medicine focused on enabling children with unusual anatomies to meet white expectations about gender and genitalia, while the racist aspects of its practice disappeared behind grand claims about human nature. Therefore, although it may sometimes be expedient to frame demands for intersex bodily integrity and autonomy in terms of human rights, that framing can signal a failure to interrogate how intersex medicine has adopted the rhetoric of humanism and how humanism itself obscures the intersections between forms of discrimination.

A HISTORY OF DISCOMFORT

It might seem that what I am moving toward in this chapter is nonetheless a humanism of feelings, an appeal to shared sentiment. Certainly, like sharing the medical articles at which my housemates winced, talking with others about the idea of bleaching babies generates a corporeal response comparable to that of medical descriptions such as *penile disassembly*—a response more immediate than the contemplation of analogies based on identity or the meaning of being human. But I shall now suggest that the relation between vicarious discomfort and the moral character of surgery is not referential. The reason for this caveat is that to posit a referential relation, whereby surgery would feel bad to others directly *because* it is bad, would be to assume that feelings can tell us the truth. Moreover, it would be to suppose a particular type of person whose interior feelings can act as a mirror for the morality of the world. The account of feelings for which I will argue is more expansive and less individualized. In a relevant essay, the critic Lauren Berlant has dissected the position of the "subject of true feeling"—a culturally constructed standpoint from which it appears possible to distinguish right from wrong on the basis of how things feel. This is a problematic construct, Berlant argues, not least because it can lead to political inaction when individuals misrecognize feeling good as evidence for the arrival of justice.[37] I agree with Berlant and have elsewhere extended this argument to critique what I call "sentimental determinism" in debates about intersex treatment.[38] Sentimental determinism is the belief that a decision about the right way to treat intersex—or indeed to demedicalize it altogether—can be reached through attention to how accounts of intersex make us feel. Sentimental determinism is not what I am proposing here.

The challenge, therefore, is to reconcile a refusal of Berlant's "subject of true feeling" with my starting contention that genital surgery not only feels bad but also is bad. Attending to the uncomfortable feelings generated in others when they hear about surgery evidently risks giving those feelings a morally referential status. However, even when the generation of uneasy feelings about surgery moves others to support the reform of existing medical practice, their feelings cannot reveal whether the right alternative to genital surgery is the patient-centered approach favored by many critics. That would be a separate debate, its outcome undetermined by sentiment. To adopt patient-centered treatment, as Chase has noted, would mean treating people with atypical genitalia by conventional standards of care rather than as exceptional.[39] Nonconsensual cosmetic surgery is certainly not standard practice in other areas of medicine.[40] Consequently, it is possible to feel bad about the fact that people born with intersex anatomies are excluded from conventional standards, but without passing judgment on the adequacy of the standards themselves or prescribing alternative standards of care. I think that this distinction addresses, to an extent, Berlant's concern about mistaking feelings for justice or injustice. It means continuing to hold open for critical reflection the interval between bad feelings about surgery and the formulation of proposals for medical improvement. To the same end, I caution against eschewing feelings altogether; Berlant's argument can be turned around to indicate that if feelings are no measure of justice, then justice is no determinant of feelings. This is to say, the morality of medical treatment for intersex does not exhaust people's feelings about it.

Far from being merely a peripheral reflection of medical practice, feelings have been central to the history of intersex—both its conventional medical treatment since the 1950s and the critiques of treatment that emerged from the 1990s on. Together, these phenomena compose a veritable history of discomfort because medical and critical discourse have had in common the aim of reducing feelings of discomfort about intersex. In Dreger's phrase, both have sought to make bodies less jarring. But traditionalists and reformists have diverged over how best to achieve this goal and for whom. In the traditional medical view, the sight of an infant's atypical genitalia has been held to cause discomfort primarily for parents, leading to a damaging lack of conviction about their child's gender, plus secondary discomfort for diaper-changing friends and relatives—triggering exclamations of dismay and subsequent gossip. Genital surgery has been claimed by traditionalists to foreclose such reactions.[41] Critics have inverted this argument by suggesting that even if atypical genitalia do cause discomfort to others, such feelings are matters of social psychology and ought therefore to be tackled through dialogue rather than through body modification.[42] As Schober stated in the late 1990s, "Early surgery makes parents and doctors more comfortable, but counseling makes people comfortable too, and is not irreversible."⁴³ A subsequent change in medical nomenclature from *intersex* to *disorders of sex development* has been recommended by some commentators on the grounds that the new nomenclature is apparently more comfortable to affected individuals than the old—that it "feels right" in its medicalizing specificity.⁴⁴ So here is another cause to reject sentimental determinism: feelings cannot guide the treatment of intersex because the management of feelings about intersex has itself been part of treatment, surgical or nonsurgical.

Adopted by medics at a major international conference in 2005, the term *disorders of sex development* was intended in part to avoid the connotations of sexual and gender identity implied by the terms *intersex* and *hermaphrodite*.⁴⁵ Yet, in turn, many critics of the replacement term have responded that it makes them more uncomfortable, not less: "I feel slimed by the shame that this new label imposes on us," Viloria has complained.⁴⁶ Objections to the revised nomenclature have coalesced around the not entirely reconcilable claims that *disorders of sex development* casts unusual bodies as inherently defective and pathologizes the identities of individuals who have such bodies. Those in favor of the term argue that it was never intended to describe an identity but rather to enable the formulation of clear standards of care where medical interventions would be genuinely useful, as opposed to traditional cosmetic surgeries that are of no demonstrable use.⁴⁷ I think, however, that the extent to which surgical procedures could ever be firmly distinguished by this criterion is uncertain. Meanwhile, some online critiques of the new nomenclature have taken the form of vituperative screeds against the integrity and motives of the nomenclature's authors, as if an appropriate response to the bad feelings generated by the term *disorders of sex development* is to make its authors feel bad, too.⁴⁸

I acknowledge that the nomenclature change has facilitated some improvements in decision-making about treatment. For instance, guidelines for UK clinicians now emphasize psychological support more strongly than genital surgery, including the provision of information about the controversy over treatment, in contrast to the traditional view that surgery can circumvent psychological concerns.[49] Yet, despite these improvements, childhood surgery remains a widespread practice, and I discuss this state of affairs further in chapter 6.[50] The dispute over nomenclature shows that responses to atypical genital anatomies continue to be polarized between feelings of comfort and feelings of discomfort, with everyone arguing that their approach is the most comfortable to the people who matter—understood variously to be patients, their families, prospective sexual partners, doctors, and so on.

But notwithstanding attempts from diverse standpoints to make intersex feel comfortable, it seems to me that just as feelings about treatment are not a simple referential mirror of treatment's morality, so too do feelings exceed the poles of comfort and discomfort. This means that feelings cannot be managed fully and finally by anyone, whether traditionalist or reformist. There are two reasons why. The first reason is that if approaches to intersex are judged wholly by their felt location between the poles of comfort and discomfort, then the body is treated as something akin to a couch—whereby the feeling of comfort would be good and inversely proportional to the feeling of discomfort. But living well in one's body does not mean feeling comfortable in the same way that one might relax on a couch. I understand the body to be one's inescapable point of view on the world, a phenomenological claim that means the world appears to oneself through bodily perception. We encounter the world phenomenally first of all. Consequently, in order for there to be

a world for oneself at all, one's perceiving body must be consti-
tutively open to impressions that are as various as the world. For
example, because my visual perception is both located within the
world and open to it, the content of my visual field changes when
I move my eyes: in a single corporeal act, I change the position
of my eyes in the world *and* change the world that appears to
me through my eyes.[51] Now, it might be very comfortable to rest
my eyes in darkness, but then the world would be lost to me
because my visual field would become monotonous. (This is not
to imply that individuals with visual impairments are cut off
from the world but to isolate one sense as a thought experiment.)
What this understanding of the body means for feelings about
intersex treatment is that unalloyed comfort would be both
unusual and undesirable. A perceiving body is not a comfortable
body; it is less narcissistic and more open than that.

THE BODY AS OBJECT

If the body's perceptual mutability must correspond to the mutability of the world in order to perceive the world at all, then the
second reason why feelings about intersex treatment exceed the
poles of comfort and discomfort is more specific. It is also more
personal. Like several others who have undergone surgery for
intersex, I have experienced genital desensitization because of
nerve damage during surgery. In my case, the damage occurred
during an operation at age sixteen—a follow-up to surgeries in
infancy—and caused a complete lack of tactile perception in
much of my genitalia for nearly a year. Genital tactility was
severely diminished for a further three and a half years such that
sexual pleasure was extremely difficult, even tedious, to obtain.
Decades after the surgery, tactility remains patchy and weak;

evidently it will never return fully. I mention this experience in some detail because I have found genital desensitization to be a singularly difficult phenomenon to communicate to others—whether in the context of giving a medical history or during sexual relations. Within the latter, its communication is not comparable to a conventional explanation of which sex acts one does and does not enjoy because sexual likes and dislikes require body parts capable of feeling comfortable (*I like this*) and uncomfortable (*I don't like that*). Indeed, one reason why desensitization is so damn inconvenient is that it, like genital surgery for intersex generally, can turn sexual relations into a cumbersome process of recounting one's medical history. This occasioning of discourse about the body causes one to fail to make sense to others as one struggles to express how it feels not to feel—to communicate not wince-inducing pain but the diminution or absence of perceptual content.

Confounding the alignment of good treatment with feelings of comfort and of bad treatment with discomfort, the desensitized feeling of no feeling is a moral injury of a strange order. Because it takes place in only one area of the body, I think that it can be understood as an injury of differentiation. This is to say, the body is experienced as being partitioned between areas with tactility and those without tactility. Previous critiques by other scholars have also asserted that medicine has a differentiating effect, but not in the manner I am suggesting here. For instance, it is true that genital surgery functions to differentiate individuals born with intersex anatomies from those born without; in the ways I have been discussing in this chapter, surgery stigmatizes rather than normalizes and thereby marks recipients of surgery as different from those who are unaltered.[52] It is true, too, that surgery endeavors to differentiate individuals in terms of bodily sex between those who are visibly male and those who

are visibly female. These are long-standing objections to the medicalization of intersex. A more recent criticism is that the term
disorders of sex development differentiates between people who have
a disorder and those who do not.[53] These various objections have
a shared interest in debunking the medical project of differentiating people from one another, whether along the lines of male or
female, surgically modified or not surgically modified, disordered or nondisordered. However, in addressing desensitization, I am interested in the imposition of differences upon
individual bodies, not between them.

The experience of lost tactility is neither a matter of contrasting oneself to others for whom sensitivity is intact nor a matter
of comparing one's state of desensitization with a prior uninjured
state. For individuals who received desensitizing surgery in
infancy, the latter comparison is impossible anyway. Rather, loss
of tactility is the ongoing experience of a contrast between sensitive areas and insensitive areas upon one's own body. At this
point, it might be objected that desensitizing surgery, unfortunate though it may be, is nevertheless discontinuous with intersex surgeries that leave nerves undamaged—in other words, that
the consequences of desensitizing surgery cannot be generalized.
This would mean that the remainder of this chapter could have
only a very specific scope. Similarly, it might be objected that
surgeries on atypical genitalia performed in infancy, whether
destructive or preservative of tactility, are discontinuous with
elective procedures on adult intersex genitalia. One might argue
that whatever undesirable effects surgery has, such effects are not
morally injurious if surgery is chosen by a consenting adult. I
think these objections would be misplaced. Consider that when
genitalia are insensate, it is as though one part of the body
remains anesthetized for surgery after the rest of the body has
awoken. The difference is one of degree, rather than of kind,

between this and surgeries that preserve tactility. Phenomeno-logically speaking, desensitizing surgery just goes on for longer: in one place on the body, the anesthetic never wears off. To put it another way, desensitized genitalia linger in a belated time zone all their own.

The significance of this phenomenological account can be amplified by drawing on a seminal essay by the feminist phi-losopher Iris Marion Young. In the essay, Young interrogates the claim that there is a particular way of "throwing like a girl." Instead of dismissing the claim as a sexist fiction, Young explains how in a sexist world certain styles of bodily movement are at once gendered and naturalized.[54] Young's argument can help to explain in more detail the crucial continuity among intersex sur-geries of all kinds. Young argues convincingly that a style of embodiment characterized by mistrust of one's body is custom-arily gendered feminine. The kind of mistrust to which Young refers is not an intellectual judgment about bodily capability but a felt sense that one's body is an unreliable conduit for one's intentions—hence, to throw like a girl is to throw badly because one feels that one's body cannot be trusted to throw at all. Under-stood phenomenologically, the body needs to disappear from one's attention when throwing an object, such that one is occu-pied entirely with the will to throw rather than with the act of throwing. Some commentators on intersex treatment have explained in similar terms the experience of parents in choos-ing surgery for their children. A newborn's atypical anatomy can appear to the parents' attention as an obtrusive object, the dis-appearance of which seems to be promised by surgery—not lit-erally (although clitoral reduction may have that aim, too) but phenomenologically in the sense of allowing a child's genitals to pass without notice.[55] However, that process concerns the pur-ported surgical differentiation of children along the lines of male and female, which is distinct from the experience of tactile partition.

I think Young's essay illuminates a different point relevant to tactility. Young suggests that if one feels pervasively unsure about the body's capacity to execute a desired action, then the act of throwing becomes one's object of attention. Young critiques the resultant faltering movement, simultaneously willful and distracted, as typically feminine. Put differently, it is the contradictory feeling of acting *on* an object in the world (the thing being thrown), while feeling that one *is* an object in the world, an obstacle to overcome in order to act. I argue that when genitalia are insensate, they are similarly experienced as part of one's body and at the same time as an object in the world. Like the feminine embodiment described by Young, the experience of desensitization is irreducibly and distractingly contradictory. Just as the act of throwing like a girl is characterized by uncertainty over the parameters of one's body in relation to the world, so too is the phenomenology of genital desensitization typified by ambiguity over where one is and where one is not. This makes clearer why desensitization cannot be conveyed in terms of comfort or discomfort: what needs to be expressed is not *I exist in that body part, and it feels comfortable or uncomfortable*, but rather *I am not sure whether I exist in that body part because it does not feel at all*. Discourses of sexual intimacy and medical history alike cannot easily accommodate body parts that belong seemingly to no one. As one former patient has put it, "Functional damage can give rise to feelings of loss of body ownership."[56] Hence, lived experience and the surface of one's skin fail to line up; the former retreats from the latter. If Young is correct that this mode of embodiment is feminine, then it is another way in which surgery genders individuals.

I suggest more broadly that all surgery for intersex is objectifying, not simply in the everyday sense of measuring the body against aesthetic norms but also in the phenomenological sense of turning a part of the body into a part of the world.[57] In this respect, there is no essential difference between whether genitalia are experienced as an obstacle to overcome *by* surgery (where surgery is experienced as successful) or an obstacle to overcome *because* of surgery (where surgery is experienced as injurious). In both cases, living in a world in which genital surgery is thinkable as a way of modifying the body leads to the objectification of genitalia. This is what Young would call the "existential phenomenology" of intersex.[58] Such is the continuity between intersex surgeries, even those that are consensual or trivial: they all involve a loss of body ownership, whether fleetingly in anesthesia or persistently in nerve damage. But that is still only part of the issue at stake.

TOGETHER IN FLESH

In this concluding section, my analysis will diverge from Young's argument because Young's interest is primarily in the inhibited capacity to affect the world. I will explore instead the inhibited capacity to be affected by others. So far I have made claims about, on the one hand, the interpersonal experience of sharing a world in which genital surgery takes place and, on the other hand, the highly personal, even isolating, experience of genital injury following surgery. I think that these divergent claims can nonetheless be synthesized to reveal something about the existential phenomenology of intersex—how the shared world in which one finds oneself determines the means by which one perceives the world. I shall show that even though an objectifying loss of body ownership is a contraction of lived experience away from the skin's surface, the perception of that loss by others is an experience that exceeds the surface of any individual's skin.

Critical readers might respond to the preceding section of this chapter by arguing that surgery of any kind, unrelated to intersex, necessarily turns into an object the part of the body on which it operates. To clarify, such an argument would refer not to a body part's physiological state after surgery but to its distracting presence in one's awareness. I acknowledge that such objectification is unavoidable, even in clearly therapeutic interventions.[59] But there is a difference. When surgery is performed on a body part such as an arm, one's capacity to affect the world is impaired by the arm's objectification: for instance, it becomes difficult to throw things. When surgery is performed on the genitalia, *one's own capacity to be affected* is acutely impaired. It is impaired because the disappearance of one's genitalia from one's awareness usually permits an experience of genitalia as transparently receptive. More precisely, it is the capacity to be affected *by others* that is disrupted by the genital objectification entailed by intersex surgery. Desensitization of the genitals limits this capacity in an especially persistent and irreversible way. What is at stake, then, is the objectification of a body part through which others can usually act on the self by virtue of that part's tactile receptivity.

It is important to explain that what I am describing is not the impaired capacity to touch and be touched, which some authors in gender and sexuality studies have valorized as exemplary of the body's constitutive openness to others. Touching and tactility are different; touching can be valued for its dissolution of the body's perceived limits only if it coincides with the interpersonal reciprocity of tactility. The diminution of such reciprocity is my concern here. Hence, I agree with the critical theorist Margrit Shildrick that bodies are existentially "leaky" in their capacity to be affected by others, but I disagree with Shildrick that such openness is exemplified by the capacity to touch and be touched.[60] One can touch and be touched without tactility—unmoved, unaroused, and even unaware of what is going on. So I think that the "leakiness" invoked by Shildrick is exemplified more accurately by the capacity to feel. By "capacity to feel" I mean neither simply emotions nor sensations because both terms would evoke a state located within an individual body. I argue more expansively that the capacity to feel is the transindividual condition of being sensible with others. This is a kind of leakiness that cannot, as Dreger put it, be jarred.

In the light of this claim about feeling, three of my earlier formulations can be revisited and unified. First, the correspondence that I posited between the body's perceptual mutability and the mutability of the world is exactly the leakiness under discussion here. As a perceiving entity, the body needs to be capable of being affected by the world. Because the world is inescapably shared, to perceive the world at all is to be affected by others—to be sensible with and among them. Accordingly, I am using the word *transindividual* now instead of *interpersonal* to emphasize that leakiness is not reducible to any given interaction between specific individuals. Second, when genitalia are objectified, they are experienced as an obstacle to overcome, but not in order to act in the same way that one might throw something. Rather, objectified genitalia are an obstruction to feeling in the transindividual sense. Specifically, the curtailment of one's capacity to be affected by others is nothing less than a dwindling of the world. The world recedes from me when I am touched without tactility. Third, because one's body comprises both sensate and insensate zones alongside each other, to live with desensitization is nevertheless not a monadic existence; some body parts remain sensible to the touches of others. Therefore, in experiencing the contrast between such zones, one is experiencing a difference in the extent to which one can be affected by others. In existential phenomenological terms, I would call that an injury of differentiation.

To lose tactility, to lose others, to lose the world—these are the same. In this regard, my argument is fundamentally unlike critiques of intersex treatment that focus on the loss of bodily autonomy.[61] I think that treatment makes individuals *too* autonomous. As Matthew Ratcliffe has written insightfully regarding some psychiatric conditions, "What distinguishes a predicament as *existentially* pathological is a particular kind of *loss*, a loss of the sense of other people or a loss of possibilities involving access to other people."[62] Consequently, there would seem to remain an absolute, unyielding division between those of us whose intersex genitalia have been desensitized by surgery and others whose anatomies are sexually unambiguous and who have not received genital surgery. This point returns my chapter to its central story. It would appear that no amount of talking with my housemates about my medical history could have expressed to them the peculiar character of the injury I incurred—irrespective of how gorily graphic I made my account. However, as I have argued, the communication of perceptual content is not the predicament here; its absence is. So in view of the analysis that I have developed in this chapter, what if it is not a *feeling* that the wincers lack, but a *lack of feeling*? To pose this question is to bring to light a surprising symmetry between my housemates and me. It is a reciprocal lack. Just as I lack feeling, the wincers lack that lack of feeling. This means that their perception of discomfort is clearly not an absence of feeling comparable to my own, but something is missing from it nevertheless precisely because it differentiates them from me. I do not feel what they feel; they feel what I do not feel—this is what separates us. Yet, strikingly, it is also something that we share, a knot of lack. Insofar as the loss of others is an existential problem, it is truly transindividual: I cannot lose others without their losing me.

If my account here sounds a little abstruse, consider that the wincing of others may signal the activation of what neuroscientists have called "mirror neurons"—areas of the brain implicated in the perception of one's movements and experience of emotions, which are also triggered (to a lesser extent) during the perception of movement and emotion in others. Some scientists have suggested that the process provides a neural basis for empathy, for it allows us to simulate the sensations that are implied by the bodies of others.[63] I suspect that the discomfiting effect of phrases such as *glans separation* and *clitoral resection* and of their accompanying illustrations coincides with the activation of mirror neurons in individuals who have not undergone genital surgery. When we feel violated at the sight of another's violated body, we are not feeling something about their violation; we are feeling violation itself. I find this neural interpretation fascinating, but with some important caveats. Simply having the right neurons does not make one empathetic: one's social and moral orientation in the world determines those with whom one empathizes.[64] This is evident from the painful decisions about treatment made by paternalistic clinicians and many parents: Ninety-five percent of parents in one study said that they would consent to surgery on their children's intersex genitalia even if tactility would definitely be impaired.[65] Moreover, I am skeptical that *empathy* is the right word for the solution to the existential problem under discussion in this chapter. The knot of lack that I have described cannot be unpicked by the "discursive use of empathy" with which some campaigners have sought to make genital cutting relevant to others.[66] Empathy means feeling something that another feels rather than something unfelt by another. Even so, the usefulness of the neural account is that when I claim that others feel what I do not feel, I mean it materially. I can no longer feel penile disassembly, but they can. Their nervous systems react where mine does not.

Another helpful term for this materiality is *flesh,* which the philosopher Maurice Merleau-Ponty once used to describe the inseparability of the perceiving body and the world perceived. Merleau-Ponty asked, "Where are we to put the limit between the body and the world, since the world is flesh?"[67] In Merleau-Ponty's writings, flesh is a foundational quality of "reversibility," whereby bodies exist in a shared world that they perceive and in which they are perceived. By this definition, objectified body parts would not be flesh because they are only perceived; they do not perceive. In such objectification, reversibility is diminished. This is another way in which the effects of intersex surgery are, as Schober put it, "irreversible." The problem is not just that they cannot be rewound in time but also that they impede the capacity of the world to fold upon itself through the convergence between perception and being perceived. Intersex surgery is therefore an injury to flesh, and when flesh is injured, our capacity to make sense with one another is impaired. Accordingly, what I have called "feelings" and what Merleau-Ponty calls "flesh" are ultimately indistinguishable; I introduce Merleau-Ponty's term here because it usefully draws attention to materiality without reducing materiality to that which can be known through science, such as the behavior of mirror neurons. I regard knowledge of the latter as valuable because it adds texture to our understanding of the phenomenal world, not because it replaces it. Most importantly, Merleau-Ponty's vision of the world as flesh indicates that lived experience does not separate us. Lived experience means living together with the medical correction of intersex variations as an injury to the flesh of the world.

With Merleau-Ponty's work in mind, reflection on the role of mirror neurons in sharing a world makes apparent something startling, even redemptive. It is conventional in neurology to define the perceptual disturbances that sometimes follow brain injuries as being sensations that are displaced from one part of an individual body to another part of the same body—for example, from the upper arm to the lower arm following a stroke. These displaced sensations are known in neurology as "referred sensations."[68] Phantom perceptions beyond the end of an amputated arm can also be understood as sensations that are referred outward into the space around the body.[69] Such phantom perceptions extend lived experience beyond the skin's surface rather than contracting from it—an expansion of body ownership, converse to its loss in the case of desensitization. But such referred and phantom sensations in a single individual have not hitherto been compared to the action of mirror neurons between different individuals. I argue uniquely that mirror neuron effects are referred sensations, too. They refer sensations *between people*, exceeding the boundaries of individual bodies and thereby leaping across flesh—in Merleau-Ponty's sense—that has been surgically injured. This original argument undoes any notion that the lived experience of intersex is purely personal. The ensuing reciprocal lack, whereby one individual's wince at surgery lacks the very lack of feeling that surgery has brought about, might be rethought not as a deficiency but as something potentially redemptive: the other feels for me—not like me but instead of me. They are affected on my behalf. Finally, then, one cannot avoid being affected by another's loss of the capacity to be affected, because we are of one flesh, as expansive as the world.

2

RUSHING TO TRAUMA

f intersex is a problem, what type of problem is it? Many intersex activists and critical commentators have challenged the idea that intersex is a problem solvable by medical treatment. In its mission statement during the 2000s, the influential Intersex Society of North America (ISNA) described intersex as "primarily a problem of stigma and trauma, not gender."[1] The society's concise and arresting claim reversed traditional assumptions about how intersex should be handled, reaching for the potent word *trauma* to express not only the panic felt by many parents and doctors in response to sexual ambiguity but also, more importantly, the impact of their panicked treatment decisions on young patients. In recent years, the human rights campaigner Daniela Truffer has highlighted "the blatant contradiction" between what Truffer calls the "lifelong trauma, loss of sexual sensation, and scars" reported by patients and the medical claim to confer normality through genital surgery.[2] The present chapter will both dismantle and rebuild such arguments about traumatization to reach a shocking conclusion. Most previous work on this topic has not defined *trauma* clearly, using it as a general term for all the negative side effects of medicalization. Typically, such effects are characterized as accidents or failures of treatment. But when the concept of trauma is used so loosely, we fail to notice that traumatic effects are not necessarily caused by treatment going amiss. I will define *trauma* more rigorously and suggest that it is not accidental but fundamental to how intersex treatment works. Diverging from Truffer, I will show that there is no contradiction between the normalizing goals of medicine and the creation of patient trauma: they are two names for the same thing. In short, this chapter will argue that the traumatization of patients is integral to the medical treatment of intersex—and therefore a prime reason why treatment, not intersex, is the problem that needs to be solved.

Even though I am going to argue that treatment is inherently traumatic, I acknowledge that medical professionals do not set out maliciously to traumatize. Indeed, some of them say that gender uncertainty is the real trauma and that the purpose of genital surgery is to avoid such trauma by providing certainty over gender assignment and development.[3] I think that this claim is indicative of a central misrecognition of trauma for gender. Medics try to avoid trauma by providing patients with a gender like any other, but they really create an event like no other—childhood genital surgery. There is a false perception among many medical professionals that the extraordinary practice of genital surgery for intersex is somehow comparable to the mechanisms of gender assignment and development for the majority of people whose anatomies are not intersex. To see such surgery as a normalizing practice by interpreting its physical and psychological outcomes as if they were ordinary is a mistake. There is nothing ordinary about having surgery in childhood to change the way your genitals look and function. I will argue therefore that the trauma of surgery is masked by the perception that surgery provides certainty over gender. Where there is trauma, medics see gender. So, as we will discover in this chapter, the

activist argument that intersex is purely a problem of trauma—
not gender—does not account for the complex relays of misin-
terpretation between trauma and gender, which operate to make
incredible surgeries seem normal and mundane. The problem is
not that there is a gap between what treatment is designed to do
and what it actually does; rather, there is a gap between what
treatment does and how it is seen. We might say that treatment
is designed to be misinterpreted. My position is that we should
take early genital surgery more literally—as painful, alarming,
and violent. It is not a normalized child who returns from the
operating theater: it is a wounded one.[4]

THE FAILURE OF CRITIQUE

I want to start with one of the most curious aspects of the debate
about intersex treatment and trauma—the fact that for many
years it did not achieve very much. It still hasn't. This is a story
of failure. I am referring not to the failure of medicine but to
the failure of criticism to achieve meaningful medical change
despite obvious deficiencies in how intersex is medically treated.
At first glance, this outcome is perplexing. If intersex is a problem of trauma, not gender, then one might assume that the role
of criticism should be to show how medical interventions that
focus on gender go and have gone wrong. Throughout the 1990s
and 2000s, activists and commentators voiced such critiques
in popular media and professional literature, across academic
disciplines, and in several countries.[5] Through scholarly arguments and patient narratives alike, we illuminated instances of
treatment going awry—genders incorrectly assigned, surgical
complications, psychological distress. Yet these efforts did not
have the impact we were expecting. Treatment largely resisted

critique; clinical practices and policies stayed much the same.[6] In looking back, there are two distinct ways to interpret this inertia. From one perspective, it is a sign that intersex medicine is uniquely wicked—brazenly unethical, stubbornly sexist and homophobic, more like female genital mutilation than evidence-based healthcare.[7] From another perspective, the lack of change is typical of medicine, which rarely advances cleanly from past mistakes to better science but is entangled in overlapping paradigms, everyday beliefs, and professional hubris.[8] Either way, medical inertia has put the task of criticism into doubt. For those of us who maintain that treatment is traumatic, our options have diminished. We could keep saying that intersex is a problem of trauma, not gender; we could stop saying it; or we could say it differently. I think it is worth saying differently.

Changing the conversation starts with recognizing that existing attempts to criticize treatment have been limited by a pervasive lack of clarity around the definition of the term *trauma* in this context. The critique of intersex medicine as traumatic often characterizes trauma imprecisely as miscellaneous psychological or emotional aspects of treatment that are aversive or harmful. For example, a twenty-two page article by a family therapist titled "Intersexuality in the Family: An Unacknowledged Trauma" (2006) does not actually define trauma; it indicates vaguely that nondisclosure "can have an untoward psychological impact."[9] An essay by another psychotherapist who is versed in trauma theory and treatment asserts that individuals with intersex characteristics have been traumatized, but it inexplicably omits to specify how.[10] Numerous others use the term *trauma* in passing.[11] In scholarship on intersex, the only analysis I have found within a clearly elaborated framework for understanding trauma is a four-page discussion in an American Psychological Association (APA) handbook on the treatment of post-traumatic stress disorder. Ironically, this short analysis appears in a chapter that frames intersex as principally a matter of gender and sex, not of trauma.[12] Both the APA handbook and the family therapy essay make cogent recommendations about psychological support for affected individuals and families, but the perfunctory use of the term *trauma* unfortunately serves to psychologize objections to medical treatment expressed by patients. That is, such objections look like the treatment's "untoward psychological impact" rather than the articulation of a principled standpoint against medicalization.[13] This has made it easy for some doctors to dismiss patient narratives as purely "public self-pity," as the intersex scholar and activist Morgan Holmes has observed.[14] Interpreted as evidence of individual psychological problems, patient narratives are liable to be discredited. As a result, many traditionalists have viewed critiques of medicine as both unreliably subjective and underrepresentative of a presumed silent majority of satisfied patients.[15]

In the absence of visible definitions, a working concept of trauma has emerged in critical discourse on intersex treatment. Critics have adopted a model of trauma organized loosely around two precepts. The first is the idea that trauma arises by omission—that it is caused by shortfalls in treatment, so that individuals are traumatized when they do not receive the support, healthcare, or information they need. In other words, to be traumatized is to lack something. For example, the intersex patient advocate Esther Morris Leidolf has argued that "increased social inclusion and exposure would help to prevent emotional trauma" but "the mental health profession has been left out of our care."[16] The second precept is the idea that trauma happens by accident—that it is at odds with the aims of treatment. Reflecting on the impact of secrecy by doctors about diagnostic and treatment information, the activist Pidgeon Pagonis has written that "in trying to *protect* me, they made me feel ashamed and isolated[,] and the stress and trauma from those surgeries left lingering severe effects."[17] This is to suggest that patient trauma is a sign that intersex treatment fails by its own measure. The working concept of trauma in critiques of medicine, then, is a kind of accident of omission. I named this the *deficit model* of trauma in my earlier essay on the subject.[18] The deficit model is a way of thinking about the relationship between intersex treatment and trauma that assumes the former is not designed to cause the latter but falls short and causes it anyway. In the words of one patient, Arlene, surgeons "built me a vagina so I could have so-called normal sex, and that left me too traumatized to ever want that."[19] In this model of trauma, which emerged in critical discourse during the 1990s and 2000s, trauma is conceptualized as a deficiency that unintentionally ensues from treatment.

ISNA's depiction of intersex in the early 2000s as "primarily a problem of stigma and trauma, not gender," was a milestone in the deficit model of trauma. It was also a tactical intervention by the most high-profile intersex advocacy group at the time to make a decisive break from medical debates around gender. By shifting focus onto "stigma and trauma," the society sought to separate critical discourse both from traditional medical claims that unusual-looking genitalia can negatively affect gender and from the alternative medical view that gender is determined by hormonal effects on the brain, not by genital appearance, which had gathered momentum during the 1990s.[20] ISNA's position was that ethical intersex patient care should not depend on figuring out the relationship between genitals, hormones, and gender.[21] I agree with the society on this point. For some other critical commentators, however, the change of emphasis to trauma and stigma seemed to close down the possibility of claiming intersex as a gender identity.[22] Certainly, in its earlier campaigning materials, such as the darkly humorous *Hermaphrodites with Attitude* newsletter and T-shirts, ISNA had argued that intersex deserves social recognition alongside maleness and femaleness.[23] Yet it had never argued directly that there ought to be more than two genders. I think that complaints about the change of focus have misunderstood the society's tactics, which were always centered on reforming medical practice. As two ISNA organizers later explained, "ISNA has never suggested people should not have the right to express their genders however they wish."[24] Reframing intersex as something other than a problem of gender enabled the society to subvert the medical premise that childhood genital surgery can yield what doctors call "appropriate gender identity development."[25] The change of focus thereby emphasized freedom of gender expression rather than the shutting of it down. By uncoupling the critique of medicine from the question of gender, ISNA highlighted that neither critics nor medics should interfere in the gender development of patients.

I diverge from ISNA not because I think intersex is really more about gender than trauma but because of how these two concepts are interlinked in treatment. Conventionally, the domains of gender and trauma appear to be orthogonal to each other: gender seems to be a matter of who you are, whereas trauma seems to be a question of what has happened to you. But what if who you are is determined by something that has happened to you—and what if the thing that has happened is childhood genital surgery? The society's shift of focus in the early 2000s made it sound as though gender and trauma were easily distinguishable—that we would know gender when we see it, we would know trauma when we see it, and we could therefore dedicate our efforts to ending "shame, secrecy, and early genital surgery," as ISNA's founder said, without needing to talk about gender.[26] By characterizing trauma as anything but gender, while simultaneously critiquing medical treatment for being all about gender, the society's maneuver had the unfortunate side effect of downplaying the traumatic qualities of treatment. To put it another way, the tactical separation between gender and trauma took for granted that medical treatment is concerned primarily with gendering patients, thus weakening the critical argument that surgical treatment is traumatic. More widely, the idea that gender and trauma are unconnected has been personified by opposing archetypes in the debate about medical reform—on one side, those patients for whom treatment yielded apparently "appropriate gender development" and, on the other side, the traumatized patients for whom treatment fell short. To date, critics have foregrounded the latter. We have never explored the possibility that these two kinds of patients may be really the same. As long as we see gender and trauma as being fundamentally separate, this possibility is hard to imagine.

To build a new critical account of treatment, I argue that we must move beyond the deficit model of trauma. A peculiar aspect of the deficit model is the fact that it stands at odds with the way trauma has been defined and theorized outside the field of intersex studies. Whereas the deficit model paints trauma as a problem of lack, the cultural and scientific history of trauma over approximately the past 150 years has not been about lack at all. Quite the opposite: it has been about trauma as a problem of excess. Rather than describing a deficiency, the term *trauma* has referred to events that cause individuals or groups to be overwhelmed psychologically—"subjected to excessive stimuli," as one psychotherapist puts it.[27] This condition of being traumatically overcome occurs in response to events that are both alarmingly sudden and abnormally macabre. The diagnosis of trauma originated during the nineteenth century in response to spinal jolts caused by railway accidents. At the time, the jolts were interpreted as causing damage to the nervous system—not simply because of the force of the impact but also because of the emotionally terrifying qualities of collisions at speeds that had been unthinkable prior to the invention of railway travel.[28] In these respects, traumatic events constitute radical and shocking departures from the perceptions, behaviors, and sensations to which individuals and groups are accustomed. They result in a breakdown of one's capacity to make sense of what has happened because they exceed all available frames of reference. The impact is what the sociologist Kai Erikson, writing in the mid-1970s, called "a blow to the psyche that breaks through one's defenses so suddenly and with such brutal force that one cannot react to it effectively."[29] As an alternative to the deficit model, then, we can think of traumatization in terms of being violently overtaken by events. In other words, the particular kind of excess that characterizes trauma is an excess of speed.

With this definition in mind, I think we need to recognize that trauma is not about what is omitted from medical treatment for intersex but about what treatment includes and the pace at which it occurs. So, instead of focusing my critique of medicine on examples of treatment falling short or going amiss, I want to address the timing, speed, and perception of treatment when it unfolds exactly as designed. This is to say, I am going to argue that the use of surgery to produce "appropriate gender development" is itself traumatic. However, before proceeding with my argument, it is important to state that what is at stake here is not a traumatic experience as such. The overwhelming impact of trauma means that events are not experienced in the usual sense because they traumatize by overtaking perception. Despite this absence of experience, trauma is also not an objective

property of events that can be detached from their psychological impact. In this regard, we might say that trauma is somehow subjective, while also striking consciousness in a way that
is different from routine and nonthreatening events so as to evade
normal perception. For this reason, there exists a long-standing
uncertainty in cultural and scientific discourse regarding whether
trauma inheres directly in events or in the impressions that events
make on those affected by them. Such uncertainty is, in fact,
characteristic of trauma. As the critical theorist Judith Butler has
written, trauma makes "the knowing of truth into an infinitely
remote prospect."[30] Therefore, through the analysis that follows
in this chapter, I will argue that intersex treatment is traumatic
not just because it means that who you are is determined by
something that has happened to you. Its power to traumatize lies
in the fact that surgery happens faster than you can perceive,
with the result that who you are is founded on something that
you do not—and cannot—know.

SUBJECTS OF SURGERY

When reflecting on the nature of surgical interventions for intersex and the claims that have been made about them, it is tempting to plot them along a historical timeline. The history of
contemporary treatment is usually narrated as a series of shifts
between three major periods—from the emphasis on rearing in
the determination of gender, which prevailed between the mid-
1950s to the 1990s, to the emphasis on the biological determinants of gender, which ascended during the mid-1990s and early
2000s, and then toward an emphasis on the interactions between
social and biological factors in the determination of gender, from
around the mid-2000s on.[31] In parallel to these shifts, there is

also a more contentious narrative that is popular with medics. This is the narrative that surgeries have become progressively less concerned with genital cosmetic appearance and increasingly concerned with genital function—in other words, that surgical interventions are now more medically necessary than ever.[32] Although it is true that surgeries have been rationalized in widely different ways since the mid-1950s, it is important to note that all such rationalizations have been largely speculative rather than based on any demonstrable outcomes from treatment. Likewise, the narrative of a move toward medically necessary surgeries has assumed the presence of a distinction between the cosmetic and functional aspects of genitalia, which is impossible to specify in practice.[33] However, that is not my quarrel in this chapter. In the context of my argument about trauma, the greatest problem with these narratives of periodization and progress is that they overstate what has changed across time and understate what has remained constant. There is something that has persisted over the years, which I want to examine in this section of the chapter. It is an enduring and simple-sounding idea that gives rise to a revealing paradox, as we will see.

The constant thread running through surgical practice is the idea that everyone should have a gender. Even as the determinants of gender have been theorized in alternating ways, the notion that we all must be gendered has remained steady. In medical discourse on intersex, this notion has the status of an apparently simple axiom. As one medical team has said, "A gender assignment should always be made," regardless of whether genital surgery is done in infancy or later in childhood.[34] In this way, the axiomatic status of gender has operated to justify surgery at any age, enabling surgery to be presented variously as something that must take place prior to gender assignment or as something that must be done after gender has been assigned, depending on the argument that medics seek to make. What is more, despite the decades-long debate over the determinants of gender, the idea that everybody should have an unequivocal female or male gender has never truly hinged on knowing how one's own gender is determined. Instead, it has been a matter of possessing the knowledge that one is gendered as a self-evident truth about oneself. Expressed in the language of critical theory, this is a question of subjectivity.[35] By *subjectivity*, I mean the ability to reflect on oneself from a perspective that is one's own, even while it is also a position within a preexisting differential structure. An example of such a structure is gender. Subjectivity describes the constitutive bind of occupying a position that is not unique to oneself (for example, as female or male) but through which one becomes intelligible as a unique subject (for example, *this* female or *this* male). Understood like this, the medical idea that everyone should have a gender is a mandate that all subjects must be gendered subjects. Subjects do not need to know how their own genders are determined but rather only to recognize themselves as being gendered and thereby to assume their individual positions.

Medical discussions of intersex have been preoccupied with ensuring that all subjects are gendered without giving serious consideration to the reason for this imperative. When reflecting on what might happen if genital surgery were not performed, medics have framed the potential consequences in terms of gender going wrong. They have evoked outcomes such as "gender uncertainty," "gender confusion," and "cross-gender identification," as though these phenomena were easy to define as well as self-evidently undesirable.[36] I think that such warnings are both vague and circular: they reiterate the importance of gendered subjectivity without actually explaining the basis for its criticality. My argument is not to complain that there is no basis at all for the insistence on gender, however. I think it does have a basis that is implicit in medical discourse. The insistence that "a gender assignment should always be made" posits the prior existence of a *desire* for gender. This desire for gender forms the implicit basis for the mandate that all subjects must be gendered; it is as if there exists a demand that can be fulfilled only by the production of gendered subjects. Yet it is strikingly difficult to work out whose desire this might be. On the one hand, medical authors have implied that the desire for gender originates in the subject—that newborns possess some sort of incipient "inside identity" to which their gender ought subsequently to conform.[37] On the other hand, the desire for gender cannot easily be attributed to any subject because it brings subjects into being through its fulfillment. If all subjects must be gendered to be intelligible in the first place, then the subject cannot predate gender. Therefore, it is hard to say whether the desire for gender originates in the subject, or the desire precedes subject formation. Furthermore, this question would not go away if we were to attribute the desire to parents and doctors instead of to patients because parents and doctors are gendered subjects, too.

I think that medical advocates for genital surgery have never properly resolved the ambiguous relationship between the gendered subject and the desire for gender. At times, they have emphasized the former, presenting surgery as being in the child's interests; at other times, they have emphasized the latter, depicting surgery as worthwhile regardless of the child's interests.[38] Some medical articles have even made both arguments simultaneously.[39] Meanwhile, complaints by several critics have centered on the idea that genital surgery tries to produce gendered subjects—a criticism that situates the desire for gender as the forerunner to subjectivity.[40] I take a different view. Instead of supposing that the gendered subject and the desire for gender can be arranged in either sequence, I want to consider the very ambiguity of their relationship. Their sequence is ambiguous, so there is a foundational uncertainty in medical practice over whether the subject is present or absent at the time surgery is undertaken. This is a complex point that warrants step-by-step explanation. We know that the stated medical purpose of genital surgery is to ensure that all subjects are gendered. We have seen that the demand for gendered subjects invokes a desire for gender as its implicit cause. We also know that it is difficult to establish whether this desire originates in the subject or somehow precedes the formation of subjectivity. Because of such ambiguity, there is corresponding uncertainty over the status of the subject at the moment when genital surgery is performed. If the desire for gender originates in the subject, then the subject must be present when genital surgery is done. In this case, the subject exists already, and surgery bestows the inner conviction of gender for which the subject already yearns. Conversely, if the desire for gender precedes subject formation, then the subject cannot be present when genital surgery is undertaken; it does not exist yet. In this alternative but equally possible case, surgery calls the subject into existence through the establishment of gender.

The practice of childhood genital surgery for intersex therefore incorporates parallel and opposing stories about subjectivity—on one side, a story that the subject is present at the time of surgery; on the other side, a story that the subject is absent at that time. To put this differently, early surgery does not answer the question of whether subjectivity precedes or follows from the modification of intersex genitalia; rather, this is the question that early surgery raises and that it leaves unanswered. In place of an answer, surgery presents a paradox in which the subject is simultaneously present and absent.[41] The paradox of simultaneous presence and absence is, I think, the only way to understand medical claims about the impact of childhood surgery on those who undergo it. To justify surgical interventions early in life, medics have made two key claims. First, they have claimed that surgery should be done urgently because young children are uniquely sensitive to their own genital appearance and functionality as well as to the ways that people react to their genitalia. Medics have said that children should therefore be shielded from the sight of sexual ambiguity and its social effects.[42] Second, they have claimed that surgery should be done urgently because young children are uniquely impervious to genital surgery—that they do not even notice that surgery has taken place, so that it can be carried out "with impunity."[43] These two claims have endured in medical discourse, even while the nature of the surgeries that they are deployed to justify has varied. For example, although most medics no longer seek to legitimize abrupt changes of infant sex in this way, they use the same arguments in defense of other surgeries to reinforce the sex that has already been assigned.[44] Together, the claim that young children possess an acute sensitivity to genitalia *and* the claim that they are insensible to genital surgery have functioned to make surgery in early childhood seem like a timely and benign intervention.

Of course, this combination makes absolutely no sense. There is no developmental basis to believe that children pass through a phase in which they are at once intensely aware of their own genitals, while also being serendipitously indifferent to surgery performed on those very genitals. On the contrary, if it were true that children are supersensitive to how their genitals look and function, then it follows that they would also be hyperattentive to genital surgery, finding it to be distressing and invasive. Similarly, if children were completely unaware of an intervention as conspicuous as surgery on their genitals, then they would be just as uninterested in their genitals under normal circumstances—irrespective of any apparent sexual ambiguity. In the latter case, concerns over gender uncertainty or confusion would never arise, and surgery would be irrelevant. So when these two claims are considered in isolation, neither one makes the case for early genital surgery. Only when the claims are considered together do they give the appearance of justifying early surgery by suggesting that there is a special period in which sensitivity and insensitivity coexist. This is where the paradoxical status of the subject comes into play, I think. For the claims about sensitivity and insensitivity to fit together, the subject of surgery cannot be purely absent or present at the moment that surgery is performed. The wholesale absence of subjectivity would mean that the child is unaware of their genitals; meanwhile, the pure presence of subjectivity would mean that the child is aware of genital surgery. The only option to reconcile sensitivity with insensitivity in defense of childhood surgery is to suppose that the subject is neither totally absent nor fully present at the time of surgery, but that it is poised in both states at once. I argue, therefore, that the opposing stories of subjectivity—as absent and present—coexist to rationalize the timing of childhood genital surgery.

I am suggesting that the paradoxical status of the subject has a crucial influence on how adults see the effect of surgery on the child. For the advocates of surgery who start from the idea that everyone should have a gender, early surgery seems to have just one impact on the child—the establishment of a gender like any other. In this respect, those in favor of surgery begin with a simple premise and draw an equally simple conclusion. But my discussion in this section of the chapter has shown that we cannot draw a straight line between these points. There is no simple truth about surgery for intersex. Rather, its interpretation is driven by a relay of assumptions and an implicit theory of subjectivity, even though clinicians do not use that word. To see surgery as simple is a misrecognition. The surface simplicity of claims about surgery and gender is propped up by the paradoxical status of the subject at the time of surgery. Consequently, I argue that this paradox is not an obstacle to surgical practice but one of its enabling factors. The paradox of the subject has sustained the practice of surgery for intersex in the face of challenges from its critics by giving such surgery a certain banality—making it seem as if the only thing that genital surgery seeks to do is to provide every child with a gender and that the provision of gender is all that surgery does. In the imagination of those who advocate early surgery, then, the paradoxical status of the subject has never been a cause for concern. Quite the reverse. It has been a reason not to worry about surgery. But in the next section, I will make a counterargument. Drawing on the definition of trauma as overwhelming, I will argue that we should be concerned indeed for the subject of surgery and the paradox that it inhabits.

DISAPPEARING EXPERIENCE

In the previous section, I theorized genital surgery for intersex from the perspective of adults who believe that it is a good idea. As we saw, those in favor of the practice maintain that its timing coincides with a period in which children are fortuitously unmoved by having their genitals cut. Based on that belief, clinicians have advocated doing surgery even as rapidly as "immediately after birth."[45] I now want to rethink these early interventions from the perspective of the patient. My view is that all children are inherently vulnerable to painful and unexpected events because of their minimal psychological and social resources, such as emotional self-regulation, social bonds, and language. The younger the child, the fewer such resources the child possesses.[46] For example, some medical professionals have suggested that surgery should be scheduled early in life to precede the growth of the patient's cognitive abilities. They draw a connection between those abilities and the "psychological risk" of anxiety and fear in response to surgery in later childhood.[47] They infer that genital surgery must be less frightening for younger patients because those patients have lesser cognitive abilities. I take the opposite view—that surgery is more frightening to such patients because they cannot anticipate or understand it. Just because younger children may not express anxiety and fear in ways that are easy for adults to interpret does not mean they are free from distress; they simply lack the ability to challenge and communicate the effect that genital surgery has on them. In this context, I think that anxiety and fear are not risks to be avoided but psychological resources that can prevent oneself from being hurt. Rather than having a serendipitous lack of impact, surgery in early childhood has a profound effect on patients whose age means that they have not acquired the means of self-defense. In short, the earlier the surgery, the less the child can do about it.

Possessing minimal psychological and social resources at the time of genital surgery, young patients are not merely unprepared for it but also ill-equipped to make sense of it afterward. Even though the adults around the child may consider genital modification to be a therapeutic intervention that guards against gender uncertainty, the child has no such frame of reference to decipher what has been done. Without a notion of what constitutes a therapeutic medical procedure—let alone a concept of gender uncertainty as a problem to be averted—the child is immersed in the sights, sensations, and ambiguities of what has happened to their body. From that perspective, the body has been inexplicably violated. It hurts. There is a brittle chemical smell, and there are pieces of strangely textured gauze. Family members and white-coated strangers are ominously preoccupied with the site of bodily violation—touching it, inspecting it, talking about it. Perhaps there is a catheter or cannula protruding from the body, baffling things that are neither me nor not-me. Contrary to the idea that genital surgery's sole effect on children is the subtle and uncomplicated establishment of gender, I am suggesting that it is an unprecedented and shocking incident for vulnerable young patients. In fact, I think that this is a more straightforward interpretation of surgery's impact than the convoluted rationalizations by those who defend its practice. For the child, I argue, surgery is an instance of what the trauma specialist Roberta Culbertson describes as "violence from which there is no escape or recourse because one's body and one's repertoire of responses are quite simply overpowered from the outset."[48] This is not a type of power that one might be able to contest, but a power that moves to brutalize the body prior to reflection or reaction. Therefore, it is untrue that children are predisposed to be temporarily oblivious of genital surgery; rather, surgery in early childhood happens at a pace that overtakes their capacity to understand it.

I contend that because early genital surgery is acutely overwhelming physically and psychologically, it is traumatic. Moreover, I think that surgery causes trauma when it goes according to plan because it is timed to coincide with the period of greatest vulnerability in early childhood. So it is traumatic by default, irrespective of any occasions on which surgery may not work as intended by doctors or may lead to medical complications. Put another way, genital surgery does not have to go wrong in order to traumatize young patients. It does that anyway. As a critic,

I am doubtful that the deficit model of trauma can account for this state of affairs because the characterization of trauma in that model—as a loss or accident of omission—does not recognize that surgical interventions for intersex are purposefully tailored to happen when patients have negligible psychological or social resources on hand to lose. If we move away from the deficit model and reconsider trauma to mean "getting more than you can handle rather than losing something that you already had," in the phrasing of the philosopher Candace Vogler, then we can see that the main problem with early surgery is not that it inflicts a loss on the patient, taking away existing resources.[49] The brutalizing impact of early surgery certainly diminishes resources such as a child's nascent sense of security and optimism, but that impact is chiefly a problem of excess rather than diminution. As one team of experts in psychotherapy for trauma victims has noted, "The irony of trauma is that recovery requires the presence of resources greater than those the victim often had in the first place," and this is especially true for children.[50] The deficit model cannot explain this aspect of trauma because it focuses on what treatment removes, withholds, or does badly. My view is that childhood genital surgery is scheduled so as to be overpowering, and that is what makes it both traumatic and efficacious in equal measure.

The analysis I am presenting here indicates that we do not need to choose between seeing genital surgery for intersex as either a traumatic failure or a precision instrument for the establishment of gender. It can be both at the same time. There is a precedent for thinking about surgery in this way, but it has received relatively little critical attention. In 1997, Tamara Alexander, an ISNA supporter, wrote a paper titled "The Medical Management of Intersexed Children: An Analogue for Childhood Sexual Abuse," which was published on the ISNA website.

It is a quietly devastating paper because of both what it says and what it does not say. Alexander frames the paper as if it were going to answer the research question of how children are affected by sexual abuse by a consideration of medical procedures that have an analogous psychological impact. Alexander proposes that early surgery for intersex is uniquely relevant to this research question because of the family secrecy and medical misinformation with which it is traditionally surrounded as well as the direct and painful genital contact that it involves. Despite this initial emphasis on understanding childhood sexual abuse, the paper unfolds in a different direction. Alexander argues that intersex surgery causes trauma in a manner that is not merely analogous to the way abuse causes trauma, but the same. Noting that triggers for childhood trauma include breaches of bodily integrity, feelings of isolation and mortal danger, and subjection to systematically misleading explanations by adults, Alexander writes that children who undergo genital surgery "experience their treatment as a form of sexual abuse, and view their parents as having betrayed them by colluding with the medical professionals who injured them." Alexander draws a parallel between statements by abusers such as *This is just a game* and assurances by parents and physicians that *I'm doing this to help you.* In both situations, there is an "emotional dissonance" between how the adults behave and how the child's body feels, causing a fracture in how the child apprehends the events.[51]

In the context of current debates about intersex, I think Alexander's paper is a major challenge to the narrative that surgical interventions are justifiable on the grounds that they are more medically necessary than ever and are no longer about genital cosmetic appearance. Alexander's pioneering argument suggests that young children cannot comprehend the violation of bodily integrity as being anything other than destructive, regardless of whether adults view the surgery as functional or cosmetic.[52] For instance, during bed rest after genital surgery, infants may undergo what one medical team has described as "four-quadrant restraint" to prevent them from twisting their catheter.[53] Tied to a bed by their ankles and wrists, these young patients do not recognize a difference between having their genitals touched by a physician or by an abuser. Accordingly, Alexander argues that the long-term psychological effects of early genital surgery and the effects of childhood sexual abuse are the same; in both cases, they are symptoms of trauma. As in abuse, Alexander writes, "the psychological sequelae of these treatments [for intersex] include depression, suicidal attempts, failure to form intimate bonds, sexual dysfunction, body image disturbance and dissociative patterns," citing multiple patient testimonies and medical case histories as examples.[54] Such symptoms function as indirect signs that something traumatic has happened. Because the original act of violence overwhelmed and evaded normal perception, only the symptoms remain. The symptoms reference an unbearable event without revealing it, encoding the origin of trauma in an opaque cluster of ongoing behaviors.[55] Culbertson has theorized that such post-traumatic behaviors constitute a belated defense mechanism: having been helpless to prevent or halt violence as it occurred, survivors develop behaviors to ward off violence in the future, but in amplified, rigid ways.[56] For example, the "failure to form intimate bonds" mentioned by Alexander can be understood as a type of self-protection, ceaselessly guarding the site where the shadow of genital surgery or sexual abuse has fallen on the body.

Yet there is also something that Alexander does not say, a critical difference between what is argued and what is implied. The most radical consequence of Alexander's argument is never expressed directly in the paper but just gestured toward. To uncover what that is, we need to retrace the shape of Alexander's argument to see where it leads. It begins with the fact that the treatments examined by Alexander are not medical interventions that go amiss, but those that go as intended. Alexander is talking about standard medical practice. It follows from this point that *all* children who receive early surgery for intersex are traumatized—including those who have no overt symptoms of trauma. In other words, when genital surgery is done in childhood, traumatization is the norm not the exception. And if that is true, then the harrowing psychological sequelae cataloged by Alexander cannot be the sole indicators that childhood genital surgery has made a traumatic impact because not all patients have those symptoms. One might be traumatized but still able to form intimate bonds, for instance. This brings us to the thing that Alexander does not say. Implicit in Alexander's paper is the conclusion that there is another postsurgical traumatic symptom more ubiquitous and mundane than all the others. It is the treatment outcome known as the *establishment of gender.* The unspoken endpoint of Alexander's argument is the radical insight that there is no separation between early genital surgeries that establish gender and those that cause trauma: there are only traumatizing surgeries that lead to different traumatic symptoms. Such symptoms may be straightforward to recognize because they mirror the aftereffects of childhood sexual abuse, or they may be more challenging to grasp. Most challenging of all is the idea that following early genital surgery for intersex, the long-term psychological effect called "gender" is really a consequence of having been traumatically overwhelmed by the brutalizing violence of standard medical treatment.

I regard Alexander's paper as an early touchpoint between intersex criticism and trauma studies that might have led commentators to an account of trauma different from the deficit model but that stopped short of drawing the conclusion that could have helped this shift to happen. Alexander never proposed that postsurgical gender is a mark of traumatization. But I will. In the previous section of this chapter, I explored how the practice of surgery for intersex is upheld by two parallel stories about children's subjectivity—one in which the subject is present at the time of early surgery and another in which the subject is absent. I showed that these stories coexist in a paradox of simultaneous presence and absence, which lets adults defend surgery on the grounds that it takes place at a time when children are at once aware of their genital ambiguity yet indifferent to genital surgery. In turn, those who advocate surgery are insistent that it has no effect on children aside from the establishment of gender, provided that it is performed early enough. By extending Alexander's argument into territory not covered by Alexander's paper, I want to upturn the claim that genital surgery is acceptable because of the subject's paradoxical status. Although it would be easy to argue that the paradoxical status of the subject is simply a fiction, that is not what I am going to say. Instead, I think the sudden violation of having one's genitals cut, the frightening experience of hospitalization, and the emotionally dissonant behaviors of adults crack the subject apart. Overtaking the child's perception and understanding, these events are unbearable and indelible at the same time. They seem to take place somewhere other than the subject, even as they happen to the subject. The result is "a break in subjectivity," as the cultural critic Hal Foster has written of trauma.[57] In this sense, the paradox of presence and absence is not a fiction at all, but a signature effect of traumatization.

I am arguing that the timing of early surgery creates the conditions for its disappearance into a break within the subject. Overrun by an event that evades normal perception, the child's subjectivity fractures into two states, which host the opposing truths that *this has happened already* and *this could never have happened*. The subject thereby registers the reality of trauma as well as its inconceivability. This is significant because it means that the subject does not arrive ready for surgery in a state of simultaneous presence and absence, sensitive to genital appearance and functionality yet insensible to genital surgery; rather, the division of the subject into a paradoxical state is an *effect* of surgical traumatization.[58] Therefore, the fundamental difference between my position and the argument in favor of early surgery is that the latter assumes the subject to be already divided at the time of surgery, so the surgical intervention has no effect on the subject aside from the establishment of gender. In contrast, I think that surgery traumatizes and divides the subject, so the apparently uncomplicated establishment of gender is a sign that the surgical event has vanished into a traumatic gap that is incomprehensible to the postsurgical subject. For the subject, this vanishing leaves behind "a fissure in the chain of events," in the words of one trauma theorist.[59] In my account, then, gender is not the absence of trauma, but the mark of a traumatic absence. On this basis, I suggest that treatment is traumatic by design because it has to traumatize the child in order to achieve its aim of establishing gender. For the adults around the child, meanwhile, the real effects of early surgery are mistaken for the formation of a gender like any other. They see the child after surgery as being anything but traumatized, interpreting the experiential gap in the child's subjectivity as a harmless result of psychological plasticity, youthful resilience, or mere forgetfulness.[60] My argument suggests that they are badly mistaken.

This original argument also carries important implications for the practice of intersex criticism. It shows that if we see gender and trauma as being separate—even opposed—then we fail to account for the ways in which they are interrelated in medical practice. Correspondingly, if we foreground patient case histories in which surgical interventions have gone manifestly wrong, then we understate the routine violence of interventions that go according to plan—including every case in which gender is established through early genital surgery exactly as intended. To omit such instances from our critique is to misrecognize the effect of surgical violation as being nothing more than the establishment of gender, which is precisely the mistake that we should expose and challenge. I think that the surgical management of intersex is traumatic every time, not traumatic by exception, and that is what we should criticize. In addition, my analysis in this chapter points once again to the limited usefulness of "lived experience" as a corrective to medical stories of intersex. In chapter 1, I showed how the idea of lived experience oversimplifies the phenomenological nature of embodiment, wherein experience can both exceed and recede from the body that appears to others. The present chapter underscores that argument from a different theoretical viewpoint. Trauma, as we have seen, is not a lived experience; it is intrinsically nonexperiential. Because the gendered subject of early genital surgery is formed by an event that was never previously experienced, the possibility of redress through attention to lived experience is quashed from the start. This subject cannot tell the truth about what has occurred because early surgery is designed to prevent that from happening. Instead, the subject sees only the untruth that the postsurgical genitals are simple markers of gender. What the subject who is gendered by surgery cannot see is that these genitals are historical artifacts, cut and crafted by unseen hands. In this way, trauma steals history away from the subject, creating a distorted relationship to time that casts lived experience—and subjectivity itself—into doubt.

AGAINST ACCELERATION

I want to close this chapter by returning briefly to the early days of the intersex rights movement. At Mount Sinai Hospital in New York in the mid-1990s, Morgan Holmes presented a paper arguing that the medical management of intersex causes "emotional trauma" and that such traumatization has been compounded by the traditional failure to disclose either the diagnosis or the nature of surgery to patients in childhood.[61] The paper was a quintessential articulation of the deficit model of trauma. Countering Holmes's argument in favor of greater transparency, some of the clinicians in the audience responded that the solution to this problem would be to do surgery even earlier. "Their idea was that the children could best be served by keeping them in complete and permanent ignorance regarding their diagnoses and surgeries," Holmes reflected subsequently.[62] In the years since Holmes gave that paper at Mount Sinai, the medical aspiration for treatments that will bypass experience has never waned. It has manifested in attempts to condense the process of normalization into a single "comprehensive genital surgery in infancy without any need for later procedures," as doctors put it.[63] Yet this idea of a one-step procedure to feminize or masculinize atypical genitalia has been a perennial feature of medical discourse on intersex. I think it has acquired a symbolic status, representing the perfect convergence of "psychological and surgical considerations," in the words of one clinician—the possibility of compressing unlimitedly complex medical interventions into an ever-smaller period.[64] In other words, it stands for the promise of acceleration. We have seen in this chapter, however, that trauma is a problem of speed and specifically a matter of the speed of wounding. When reconsidered through the model of trauma that I have provided here, "comprehensive," single-stage childhood surgeries deepen and broaden the wounding of the body. They go farther, faster.

One-step surgeries are not the only manifestation of the medical aspiration to bypass patient experience, however. Even when one-step surgeries are intended to be comprehensive and final, complications often mean that additional surgeries are performed nevertheless.[65] So in an effort to foreclose the experience of surgical treatment once and for all, some medics have prescribed a steroid named dexamethasone to expectant mothers, which can avert the development of fetal intersex characteristics entirely.[66] Although dexamethasone affects only certain types of genital atypicality, its use for this purpose exemplifies how gendered subjects are formed by medical interventions that they can never know. The prenatal administration of dexamethasone may make the overt violence of genital surgery redundant, but I think that in doing so it transforms the fetus's entire body into a clandestine wound. With prenatal dexamethasone, the medical management of intersex recedes from a one-step process into what we might call a "nonstep" process, about which there is seemingly nothing to disclose—if, of course, one assumes that infusing a fetus with steroids to manipulate genital anatomy counts for nothing. I argue, therefore, that the acceleration of medical treatment for intersex cannot prevent trauma. In the gendered subject of dexamethasone, whose genitals look unremarkably typical, the nonexperiential trauma of medical treatment reaches its final form. As treatment speeds toward an interval of zero duration, the subject's relationship to time becomes more and more distorted—shaped by an intervention in an unknowable past, an incomprehensible medical history. I think that the answer to the problem of trauma is not to go faster, but to stop.

3

HAUNTED ATTACHMENTS

ttachments of all kinds pose a challenge for those of
us who would reform intersex medicine. It is common-
place to complain that treatment interferes with the
development and expression of gender and sexuality, as though
the defining problem with medical interventions were the prevention of individuals from being or becoming truly themselves.
According to such complaints, intersex medicine is objectionable not because it is poorly executed but because it has a con-
straining effect on individuals even when it is technically well
done. Typically, the complaint is put in one of two ways—that
genital normalization spoils an individual's "authenticity" in the
present or spoils their "right to an open future" beyond childhood.[1] Sometimes the two claims are put together to say that a
person's authenticity in the present has been blighted by an earlier failure to keep open their future, most especially by irreversible surgery in infancy. For instance, the authenticity of one's
gender and sexuality in adulthood could be undermined if the
body parts on which they are premised were secretly surgically
constructed or even removed years earlier.

The complaint of inauthenticity can imply that personhood
generally or gender and sexuality specifically would be more

authentic if they developed outside the influence of other people.[2] I am unconvinced that this is the case, though, because I do not think there is a simple polarity between self-determination and external influence. We cannot evade the influence of others; to be parented at all is to be subject to uncountable particularities that are not one's own, so that one's future is never wholly open, and one's self is never simplistically authentic.[3] I agree with the psychologist John Bowlby, seminal theorist of attachment, that dependence and independence are complementary.[4] Because personhood is relational, its measure is never the purity of our self-determination, now or in the future, but the quality of our attachments to others. For example, the feelings that parents have about their child's genital anatomy can shape the quality of their attachment to their child. When those genitals are confusing or unusual, parental feelings are rarely positive: as medical traditionalists and reformists alike have observed, the birth of a sexually ambiguous child can prompt parents to feel apprehensive and distressed.[5] So, in this chapter, I want to explore what happens when parents become attached to a child whose anatomy makes them afraid.

Some readers might interject that this discussion starts from a false premise. They might say that parents who opt for traditional intersex treatments do so because of weak or nonexistent attachments to their children—that such parents simply do not care. My interpretation of these parental decisions will be different. Diverging from other accounts of attachment formation in families affected by intersex, I am going to argue in this chapter that parental behavior is indeed animated by strong attachments, but ones that are bad. I will go on to theorize these attachments in terms of fear, exploring how parents are afraid that their child's anatomy has transgressed a social prohibition on intersex. Combining developmental psychology with psychoanalytic theory, I will then show how this prohibition is elaborated and transmitted through the language with which parents talk to their children. Finally, I will propose that bad attachments impair children's capacity to remember the genital characteristics that they had prior to treatment. This impairment of autobiographical memory clouds the authenticity of affected individuals in a way that is neither a straightforward loss of autonomy nor a foreclosure of the future. Rather, I will argue that intersex medical treatment blights one's sense of a past shared with other people and so distorts the authenticity of one's relationships with them.

THEORIZING ATTACHMENTS

Although theories of attachment rarely receive sustained consideration in the literature on intersex, traditionalists and their critics hold sharply contrasting positions on the connection between medical interventions and attachment. They disagree over whether treatment for intersex facilitates or impedes attachment formation. Summarizing the traditional position for a landmark policy statement in 2006, a group of medical professionals and patient advocates reported a widespread conviction that cosmetic genital surgery in infancy "relieves parental distress and improves attachment between the child and the parents." In this traditional view, attachments are good, and a benefit of treatment is that it strengthens attachments that would otherwise be weak or nonexistent. This is a belief, however, not a research finding. Though the policy statement cautioned that "the systematic evidence for this belief is lacking," the belief remains popular.[6] For example, in the years following the statement many clinicians have continued to insist that "we believe early operations improve the attachment between a child and its parents," but without offering any supporting evidence; and the parents of genitally atypical children have routinely supposed that they are "better placed to parent, protect and bond with their child" by the cosmetic modification of the child's genitalia.[7] The traditionalist standpoint therefore implies that parents do not need to be attached to their child in order to make good treatment decisions because treatments enable such attachments to form. Moreover, according to this view, the more genitally normal a child looks after treatment, the stronger the ensuing attachment with the parents is likely to be.

Reformists of intersex medicine disagree. They argue that medical interventions should not be decided by parents whose attachments are weak or absent. For instance, the patient advocate Anne Tamar-Mattis has contended that even if parents fail to form attachments with intersex children prior to medical treatment, that is no grounds for treatment to proceed. By Tamar-Mattis's account, parents who lack such attachments cannot empathize with their children's interests in order to choose appropriate treatments in the first place.[8] In this regard, the reformist standpoint acknowledges that attachments between parents and their children can be obstructed by the presence of atypical genitalia. Yet reformists draw from this insight a different conclusion from traditionalists, interpreting parental approval of surgery to change genital appearance as symptomatic of a failed attachment, not as its remedy. As the philosopher Ellen Feder has written, "In focusing on genital appearance, rather than on the experience of the child, the mother fails to identify with her child" and thereby "puts both her child and her relationship to her child at risk."[9] Feder's theory is reflected in one mother's recollection that early surgery on her baby meant that she "never ever felt maternal" because "you can't form a proper bond with a baby that people are just fiddling with constantly."[10] Whereas traditionalists cast treatment decisions as good when they enable attachments, reformists argue that good treatment decisions are those driven by bonds that preexist treatment—and the decision not to do cosmetic genital surgery is a sign of a strong attachment.

Despite these differences between their positions, commentators in the debate over intersex medicine agree that attachments between parents and children are beneficial. Tamar-Mattis's suggestion that parents who lack attachments ought not to decide on treatments for their children implies that the presence of such attachments would conversely allow consideration of their children's best interests. Equally, when clinicians say that early cosmetic surgeries strengthen attachments, they assume that such a change would be a desirable outcome. Starting from the common principle that attachments are self-evidently good, traditionalists and critics of medicine divide over whether this means that attachments follow from treatment, in the traditional view, or that treatment follows from attachments, in the reformist view. The direction of causality may differ between the two accounts, but each side argues for their preferred treatment decision—surgery or no surgery—on the basis of its relevance to attachments. My view is that these arguments work only if one presumes that attachments are inherently beneficial. It may sound like a commonsense presumption. However, when attachments are so defined, commentators on all sides struggle to explain how parents who are attached to their children can make bad choices, whatever a given commentator regards a bad choice to be. All commentators perceive attachments with bad outcomes to be intrinsically contradictory. Yet by theorizing attachments more carefully, I am going to argue that attachments can indeed be bad. Drawing on the work of Bowlby, I will reveal that there is no contradiction here.

Bowlby's writings on psychology recognized that attachments, including those between parents and children, are not always beneficial. Bowlby theorized that attachments originate in "the attraction that one individual has for another individual" and that these "affectional bonds" can move individuals to protect one another. For instance, an adult can be moved to protect a baby. However, Bowlby noticed that it is also possible to feel affection without behaving protectively. A bond that does not inspire protective behavior is still an attachment, according to Bowlby: it may not provide safety, yet it may be rich in affection all the same. It follows that the lesson we learn from our experience of attachments is not indiscriminate dependence on others, but a more subtle accomplishment—the discernment of when trust should be given and received. Bowlby regarded the development of this discernment as an incremental process rather than a one-off event. It is the mental construction of "working models" of those to whom we are attached. For Bowlby, a working model of an attachment figure encapsulates the history and expectations of another's behavior, providing a mental framework for whether and when to trust them. Crucially, such a model can represent an attachment figure as being untrustworthy as well as benign; protective figures are not the only ones who are modeled in this way. In a working model, then, another person may be characterized as unreliable or even hostile on the basis of past interactions. Bowlby argued that one's own self is the subject of a working model, too, which depicts for us the role we play in relation to others.[11] This particular model lets us navigate the expectations placed upon us, for it indicates our trustworthiness. If one behaves inconsistently toward people, then such behaviors reflect and intensify a working model of oneself as an unreliable attachment figure. In summary, Bowlby's theory takes seriously the function of disappointing and damaging attachments in how we learn about ourselves and those around us.

In work on families affected by intersex, the widespread assumption that attachments are purely beneficial is both a cause and a consequence of the lack of scrutiny that attachments receive. For many writers, it is as if the presence or absence of an attachment were the only thing to be known about it—as though the weight of its presence were synonymous with the extent of its beneficence. Bowlby's account, however, shows that attachments are more complex, so they should be approached with critical curiosity. Even supposing that existing parental attachments were intensified by infant genital surgery, that would not automatically turn parents into protective or trustworthy attachment figures after surgery. I think the reverse is more likely: in the child's working model of the parents, the child would register the fact that parental affection is dependent on the cutting of one's body. This would place in doubt the parents' reliability as attachment figures. Put another way, if it were true that parents experienced a sudden deepening of affection toward their child following genital surgery, then the very suddenness of that change would introduce uncertainty into the child's representation of the parents. The change would destabilize the child's ability to predict future parental behavior: the child may fear that the parents' affection will be withdrawn again with equal suddenness. Correspondingly, the child's working model of the self would register a failure to have been adequate for the parents, rendering the child's own reliability doubtful, too.[12]

Given the inability to elicit emotional consistency from these key attachment figures, the child would lack a model of themselves as trustworthy.

With this analysis in place, I argue that treatment for intersex does facilitate attachments, but they are bad ones. My position on this matter is not the middle ground between traditional and reformist views, but a radical reinterpretation of both. Where clinicians claim that early operations improve attachments, I think that this means such operations amplify bad attachments rather than transform them into good ones. Where Feder proposes that treatment leads to a failure by mothers to identify with their children, I disagree that the problem is the wholesale absence of attachments; rather, it is the presence of attachments *other than* benign parent–child identification. In fact, psychologists have identified three bad forms of attachment through studying families in which parental trust and protection are in doubt: the avoidant, ambivalent, and disorganized attachment styles.[13] The avoidant style is the most consistent, whereby children respond to untrustworthy parents by appearing to be unemotional and therefore autonomous. In the ambivalent style, children are more overtly preoccupied with their parents yet are unsettled in their presence, exhibiting an awareness that the parents may behave unpredictably. The disorganized style is chaotically disjointed, indicating that children cannot anticipate their parents' behavior at all. Importantly, attachments in all these styles can be intense and persistent.[14] Their intensity and persistence do not mean they are beneficial, though. It also does not follow that expediting such attachments by performing cosmetic genital surgery would be a good idea.

By considering the different forms that bad attachments take, I think we can understand how intersex medical treatment is damaging not when attachments fail to form but when they take root. I want to focus on the avoidant and ambivalent styles in particular. Psychologists in fields beyond intersex studies have observed that "children whose caregivers tend to be emotionally unavailable or intermittently responsive" often form attachments in the avoidant or ambivalent styles.[15] One might imagine that parents would try to prevent this, but, surprisingly, parents whose children have undergone genital surgery for intersex point to their own unavailability and intermittent responsiveness as being *positive* outcomes of the surgery. Describing a state that I would characterize as emotional unavailability, one parent said of their child's genital atypicality, "We don't even talk about it anymore. It's just not an issue for us anymore, you know. It's been repaired, and that's it."[16] These remarks express withdrawal ("we don't even talk about it anymore") and discontinuity ("it's been repaired, and that's it"). They also display profound disregard for whether the child would benefit from talking about what has happened—a detail to which I will return later in this chapter. Another parent reported behavior that I would characterize as intermittent responsiveness, recounting that "it comes and goes in waves with us definitely . . . he has his surgery and everything and it's 'oh my gosh, it's kinda real again.' After he recovers from the surgery he's just, you know, he's our normal little boy, doing his stuff."[17] When parental responsiveness is withdrawn or irregular in the ways shown in these comments, I think children are likely to adopt either an avoidant attachment style that mirrors parental unavailability or an ambivalent style that expresses wariness of future shifts in parental affection ("it comes and goes in waves"). Poised in a state of vigilance, such children may anticipate that additional genital cutting will be demanded of them to maintain parental attention and care. This discussion shows, contrary to Tamar-Mattis, that intense attachments between parents and children can act against children's best interests. It also raises the question of whose interests are really served by surgery for intersex: To whom does it matter whether a child is made into a "normal little boy," if not the child? I will turn to this question in the next section and examine the key role played by other people in the attachments that form between parents and genitally atypical children.

TRANSGRESSING THE WORLD OF OTHERS

The notion that parents just want their child's genitalia to look as normal as possible is both a cliché and a puzzle. To those of us who advocate change in the medical treatment of intersex, it seems incredible that parents who care about their children could sanction the painful and frightening removal of healthy genital tissue on the grounds of appearance alone. To explain this apparent contradiction between care and harm, it is customary to define the problem as one of medical influence. By defining the problem in this way, arguments against traditional treatment avoid criticizing parental behavior on the basis that the families of children with sexually ambiguous anatomies are steered by doctors into making treatment decisions that they would not otherwise choose.[18] Critics therefore lament that families are misled by doctors who, though powerful, lack the expertise or understanding—such as dedicated training in psychology, gender, and sexuality—that would enable them to provide appropriate advice.[19] Consequently, critics challenge the actions of parents only indirectly through objections to the advice on which they act. Based on my discussion in the previous section, however, I regard this view of parents as overgenerous. When our critical attention centers on the quality of medical guidance received by parents, we fail to tackle candidly their role in choosing invasive and irreversible treatments, including infant genital surgery. (I acknowledge that a minority of parents do not choose such surgery; I admire them, and this discussion is not about them.)[20] In this section, I am going to highlight how many parents agree to surgery in the absence of clear therapeutic goals and do so even after they have been warned by doctors of numerous likely complications. I will propose that parents are driven neither by their own carelessness toward their children nor by poor advice from medics, but by a sense of something that comes from other people.

Swift parental consent to genital surgery could be interpreted as a means by which parents can avoid conversations about their children's potential sexual function, which they may find emotionally challenging.[21] This avoidance is probably a contributing factor in treatment decisions for many families. One support-group leader has suggested more broadly that the focus on gender identity throughout the field of intersex medicine may be a smokescreen for sexuality—a means to rationalize genital cutting without making direct reference to future sexual capacity.[22] In other words, the idea that genital surgeries facilitate gender development may serve to shield both parents and medics from uncomfortable discussions about the lifelong implications of having atypical genitalia. After all, as the scholar Samantha Murray points out, "most parents do not imagine the experience of having a child as a process that will require them to think about the limitations and problems of a dimorphic sex system." Yet Murray goes on to infer that parents respond positively when their assumptions are challenged in this way—that their child's ambiguous sex anatomy prompts them to question their existing understanding of sexual dimorphism.[23] I disagree. If we look at what parents affected by intersex actually say about their treatment choices, it becomes clear that they neither speak frankly about sexuality nor think critically about sexual dimorphism. On the contrary, many parents are unashamedly unthinking. For example, one parent has recalled that "we really never had to make a decision" about treatment because "the doctors told us what was gonna need to be done." Likewise, another said of clinicians that "anything they asked for or wanted to do, I was ok with it."[24] Indeed, parents seem strangely compelled to avoid thinking carefully about the choices they make; a family with two genitally atypical children opted for surgery on their second child even after multiple complications had arisen from surgery on the older sibling, and they admitted afterward to regrets about the second child's postoperative infertility and potential nerve damage.[25] That is not thoughtful parenting.

In short, when reading accounts of parental decision-making, I am struck that for many there is, as they attest, "never any question" about whether surgery should take place.[26] Feder has attributed this lack of careful thought to the indirect influence of doctors, suggesting that although decisions are "not made *for* parents," they may be "made *through* them."[27] Certainly, some parents recall that doctors casually assume family agreement to traditional treatments and never offer alternatives.[28] Yet, interestingly, by far the most common explanation given by parents, when asked, is that treatment decisions originate with neither themselves nor doctors. Rather, they attribute to *everyone else* a prohibition on intersex that demands its surgical eradication. I want to take seriously this perceived prohibition because I think it is a central feature of the parental experience of intersex. For instance, the reasons given by a range of parents for their consent to infant genital surgery include the impression that "you have to conform to the way that the public says you should be," the feeling that "society is a big issue here," and the conviction that a requirement for genital normality is "the way our world works."[29] Public, society, world—in all three cases, parents present *someone else's* intolerance toward their child's body as the parents' problem to solve by surgery. This sense of a prohibition that is not one's own is especially clear in one mother's remark that to choose genital surgery means that "you go with the majority, you go with what you think is right."[30] At first glance, she is describing two very different imperatives—adopting a majority view and holding a view of one's own. But the slippage in her comment between the two imperatives exemplifies how parents experience a prohibition on intersex as belonging to anyone other than themselves: here, the perceived "majority" view in favor of surgery determines "what you think is right" because, circularly, it is the view of the majority. By this choice of words, the mother avoids describing herself as a member of the very majority whose view she upholds.

Rather than parents' decisions being driven by doctors or by a reluctance to talk about embarrassing topics, I contend that families feel moved by a prohibition on intersex that seems to originate elsewhere. When parents insist that genital surgery must be done because allowing a child to grow up without surgery would cause a "whole childhood" of being "socially ridiculed," I think it does not matter whether other people would really behave in the grievous way that parents imagine.[31] It matters that parents feel as though the majority of people would do so. At work here is something more nuanced than a straightforward failure by parents to imagine that the social world can accommodate children with atypical sex anatomies. As it turns out, the very parents who describe intersex as being forbidden by others can quite readily imagine circumstances in which intersex would be accommodated. Scenarios for which parents say that normalizing surgery would be unnecessary include "if people accepted that everybody's different," "if we lived on a deserted island," and "if you could say you could be male, female or something else."[32] I recognize that to a degree these statements are straw arguments against medical reform: no critics of surgical treatment propose that the only alternative to genital normalization would be to assign all affected children to a third sex or that families ought to live in seclusion. The imaginary scenarios perform a more subtle function than straw arguments, however. By drawing a line between what parents call "an ideal world," which is tolerant but does not exist, and "the way our world works," which is prohibitive but exists purely among other people, parents cast both the tolerance and the prohibition of intersex as having nothing to do with them.[33] This relieves them of responsibility for their actions and at the same time masks their own social situation by implying that the world stops where the family begins.

I am arguing that the twin concepts of a tolerant ideal world and a prohibitive real world interlock and operate together. On the one hand, they foreclose the prospect of tolerance toward intersex in reality. On the other hand, they obscure the idealized nature of its prohibition. The effect is to make the prohibition on intersex seem incontestable and traditional surgical treatment inevitable. This manner of thinking enables parents to act on the basis that, as they say, "we really never had to make a decision." It follows from this analysis that parental assent to normalizing surgery is a way of prohibiting genital atypicality on behalf of other people. The authenticity of parents' actions is doubtful, therefore. Parents maintain what critics have called "conformity with and obedience to the duty of the norm," but rather than perceiving that to be a personal or universal principle, they experience it as a socially contingent obligation.[34] So although it is true that doctors hold professional power during medical consultations and even that their advice to parents is often slanted in favor of surgery, it is true, too, that parents carry into every consultation and treatment decision a tenacious belief that the majority of people in society abhor intersex. For such parents, the argument that they may be acting under excessive medical influence is incidental because they already profess to be influenced by a whole world of others—to be going "with the majority." This helps to explain why, despite decades of criticism, medical practice has been so resistant to change: most parents have not thought to ask for anything different.[35] I suggest, then, that parents are unthinking not by accident but precisely because of their presumed obligation to others for whom they imagine that intersex is intolerable. When they come to choose treatments, they feel simultaneously that *I must do this* and that *this is not my doing*—they feel, in other words, inauthentic.

In turn, these parents anticipate a lack of authenticity in their children. This is no surprise to them; they intend it. When asked about their decisions, parents explicitly juxtapose early surgical interventions against letting their child be "accepted for who she is," as one parent said, and against allowing their child to "decide for his self," in the phrasing of another.[36] In such comments, parents openly contrast surgical normalization to acceptance and self-determination. The contrast serves to cushion parents from criticisms that their treatment choices stifle their child's personality. In the introduction to this chapter, I noted that such criticisms usually center on an individual's authenticity in the present or on the openness of their future. In starkly direct admissions, parents acknowledge that treatment does exactly what critics say. They absorb the criticism that treatment lessens a child's authenticity in the present by asserting that their child already cannot be "accepted for who she is." They absorb, too, the criticism that treatment would lessen a child's authenticity in the future by mandating that their child will never "decide for his self." To tell such parents that their actions cause inauthenticity in their children would be to tell them what they already know. For them, however, a lack of personal authenticity is the expected result of medical interventions rather than cause for medical reform. To me, regardless of the disarming simplicity of these parental admissions, something more complicated is happening. I see a curious symmetry between the inauthenticity that parents express in their submission to a prohibition that belongs to other people and the resulting inauthenticity of their children. Both generations in this relationship lack authenticity. Just as the former feel moved to act in ways that are not their own, the latter become someone besides themselves. We might put it that the personhood of the genitally ambiguous child is tied to the experience of the parents. This suggests that a form of transmission occurs through the attachments that join family members to one another, which I want to theorize next.

FAMILIES IN FEAR

Over the first half of this chapter, I have argued for the relevance of attachments to the medical management of intersex and for the salience of a perceived prohibition on intersex to parental decisions about treatment. It is now time to consider whether attachments directly play a part in treatment. For example, when genital surgery is used to make an ostensibly "normal little boy," to what extent do intergenerational attachments shape the child's apparently normal gender identity? Given my claim in chapter 2 that early treatment is traumatizing in its swiftness and incomprehensibility, it remains to be seen whether surgery itself has anything to do with gender in the everyday sense. Clinicians and parents often insist that genital appearance affects "psychosexual development" and that infant surgeries "benefit the development of gender identity in childhood," yet they never detail how.[37] A plausible interpretation in terms of attachment would be to say that children who undergo treatment identify with the gendered behavior of their parents. Identification, in this context, would mean an attachment so intimate that an individual adopts the qualities of somebody else. In threatening situations, identification with a perceived aggressor can be a means to gain control and escape passivity.[38] If the purported surgical establishment of gender is really the traumatization of patients, then identification by children with their parents might explain how gender is produced by treatment after all. Simply put, surgery could frighten children into becoming like their parents, who are the apparent source of the threat to the child's bodily integrity. By this mechanism, gendered behaviors exhibited by parents could be internalized to become gendered behaviors by children. Moreover, the same behaviors in children could be interpreted by adults as a successful treatment outcome. This idea of gender as a defensive identification pries open an important distinction between the attribution of treatment outcomes to genital appearance and their attribution to surgery. If traditionalists are right that changing a child's genital appearance affects gender development, that outcome may be not because the child's genitals look different after surgery but because cosmetic genital surgery hurts and is scary.

In several respects, this account of gender is compelling. As an explanation for the impact of early medical treatment, it emphasizes the significance of others to the self. It suggests how treatment ingrains inauthenticity in children through the internalization of parental behavior as if it were the children's own. One might ask why children would perceive their parents to be the source of the threat that triggers identification rather than those adults who perform the surgery. Both perceptions are possible, and children may certainly internalize the gendered behaviors exhibited by medical staff, too. But it seems to me more tenable that children would attribute the adverseness of surgery to the attachment figures on whom they depend rather than to clinicians whom they see rarely, if at all, because of anesthesia. Nevertheless, despite the possibility that gender acquisition is an identification induced by the fright of medical treatment, that is not the argument I am going to develop in the remainder of this chapter. This is because I think that gender is not really the most conspicuous feature of parental behavior witnessed by children who undergo medical interventions. Instead, I think that the feelings and actions displayed by parents to children during treatment for intersex are far more noticeably about the *prohibition on intersex itself.* We should remember that these people are straining desperately to eliminate intersex from their families, weighed down by their professed duty to the public, society, the world. It is the perceived social abhorrence of their child's sexual ambiguity that consumes them more than the exhibition of their own genders. With that in mind, my goal from this point in the chapter is to analyze how affected children acquire from their parents not gender but subjugation to a prohibition. Turning from the child's fear of surgery to the parents' fear of the child's anatomy, I will show how the prohibition on intersex is transmitted between generations. To advance my analysis, I will draw on psychoanalytic theory.

The psychoanalyst Maria Torok once discussed a case in which a mother refused to touch her four-year-old son's penis at bath time. I am aware that psychoanalysis is, of course, famously preoccupied with genitals. Nonetheless, one could say the same about intersex medicine, so I believe psychoanalysis is useful in this context precisely because it has things to say about how parents and children think and feel about genitalia. In the case discussed by Torok, the son asked his mother why she would not touch his penis while powdering him after his bath. The mother told him that it would be "dirty" to do so. Torok points out that the mother rehearsed on the child a "prohibition to which she herself had been subjected previously"—namely against masturbation. But rather than telling her son not to masturbate, she expressed instead an oblique "fear of the genitals" by incongruously saying that it would be dirty to touch his clean penis. The case illustrates how a prohibition from elsewhere, here against masturbation, can provoke parents to exhibit fear. As Torok writes evocatively, the mother was moved to "tremble before another person" who had proscribed masturbation for her, yet that person was absent from bath time and a stranger to her son.[39] I think this case indicates how a child with no reason to fear one's own genital anatomy could be subjected to somebody else's prohibition on intersex. Believing that between their sexually ambiguous child's legs lies something despised by all of society, many parents react to the child with "great apprehension" and "psychosocial stress," report clinicians.[40] One mother even called her newborn's genitals "disgusting" and was observed to turn pale, tremble, and begin crying upon being told by doctors that the child's sex was uncertain. Like the mother at bath time who trembled before someone who was not there, the trembling woman who termed her baby's intersex genitalia "disgusting" exclaimed that she did not know what she would tell "people on the street" about the baby's sex.[41] In this way, people whom a child has never met intrude into parental speech and behavior, binding the child to a prohibition through the parents' fears.

The prohibition to which parents of genitally atypical children imagine themselves to be obligated requires that even though they know about intersex in their child, they keep it secret—hence the comment by one parent that "we don't even talk about it anymore" following surgery. After treatment, then, there is a divergence between parental knowledge and parental speech, just as the mother at bath time said one thing but feared something else. When parents select medical treatments that purportedly make intersex characteristics go away, they remain aware that their child was born sexually ambiguous. Yet they endeavor to conceal from their child the fact that the child's genitals were ever transgressive.[42] This creates a gap between what the parents of a postsurgical child say (for example, "he's just, you know, our normal little boy") and their secret knowledge (he's not a boy, he's not normal). They withhold this information from their child on the premise that the child will be ignorant of the anatomy that existed at birth. It is traditional in intersex medicine to assume a directly proportional relationship between disclosure by parents and the knowledge held by children. If disclosure and knowledge are proportional, then a child to whom nothing is disclosed knows nothing at all about intersex, despite having experienced life with an intersex anatomy before treatment. Writing on the family dynamics of secrecy, the scholar and psychoanalyst Esther Rashkin has remarked that families with shameful or disturbing histories not only protect the "unspeakable content of the secret" but also "suppress any desire to know or understand its origin."[43] In Rashkin's terms, parents suppose that by keeping intersex "unspeakable," their child will neither learn anything from them nor have any residual knowledge of the intersex characteristics that predated treatment. In short, the perceived prohibition on intersex demands that parents know about intersex but do not say it and that children experience intersex but do not know it. To keep intersex secret, both these demands must be met.

I argue that all such efforts to maintain that intersex never existed are contradictory. This is because the traditional approach to managing intersex relies on two incompatible models of how the mind works. On the one hand, for parents to know about their child's sexually ambiguous anatomy but not to talk about it, there must be a distinction between knowledge that is consciously expressed (such as "he's a normal boy") and another type of knowledge that is mentally present but hidden (such as "he's not a normal boy"). On the other hand, for children to have experienced intersex but not know about it because their parents do not talk about it, there can be no distinction between different types of knowledge; here, information that is not consciously expressed is simply unknown. In the first of these two models of the mind, there is an unconscious. The concept of an unconscious is necessary to account for information that is known by an individual but staunchly withheld or even denied by that individual. In psychoanalytic terms, we would say that such knowledge is repressed—it is "unspeakable content," as Rashkin says.[44] The second model of the mind, contrastingly, does not feature an unconscious. In that model, an individual's knowledge is coextensive with their conscious awareness and extends no further. Nothing is repressed, for there is nowhere to repress it. The absence of the unconscious is necessary to explain how an individual could lack knowledge of having experienced life with an intersex anatomy prior to surgery: instead of hidden knowledge, there is just an absence of knowledge. In place of unspeakable content, there is no content. In these ways, the traditional approach to intersex relies on the contradictory coexistence of a model of the mind in which the unconscious exists and a model in which there is no unconscious.

It is tempting to challenge the nondisclosure of information about intersex by arguing for more disclosure. All the same, that would leave unchallenged the idea that there is a directly proportional relationship between what parents say and what children know. I am more interested in how those who advocate the medical elimination of intersex attempt to resolve the contradiction between their two models of the mind. Their attempted resolution is to say that young children are amnesic. They claim that a "psychological benefit" of early surgery for intersex is that the surgery predates "the infant's inability to form long-term memories."[45] For traditionalists, such amnesia is beneficial because it means the child will be "unaware of the ambiguity" that existed at birth.[46] The absence of intersex from the child's memory fulfills the imperative on families to maintain that intersex never existed. Now, I recognize that there is some evidence from developmental psychology to corroborate that younger children find it harder than older children to recall events from the preceding two years.[47] Yet such research is never cited by physicians who write on intersex.[48] Proponents of intersex medicine also overlook competing findings by psychologists that some individuals can recall events that occurred at age two or younger and that recollection itself varies over time. For instance, during childhood individuals may not recall early life experiences, but they may do so in adulthood.[49] In the traditional literature on intersex, childhood amnesia is treated as a simple precipice beyond which individuals have no knowledge of what has happened to them. Clinicians differ over where they suppose that precipice to be, sometimes placing it as high as age five.[50] I find this assertion highly dubious because it implies either that children remember nothing whatsoever from their first five years of life or that they somehow fail to recall only information about their genitals. Neither possibility is credible.

Nevertheless, through the assumption of childhood amnesia, traditionalists appear to reconcile their two models of the mind. Claiming that children are amnesic until a certain age, whenever that may be, enables them to suppose that the mind is absolutely different between generations. They hereby assign to children a model of the mind without an unconscious and to parents a model of the mind with an unconscious. However, in the final section of this chapter I will present an alternative argument: I shall contend that the presence of a family secret means that the generations are joined rather than separated by the unconscious.

AN UNCONSCIOUS INHERITANCE

I am going to show that the unconscious repression of intersex by parents stops children from knowing their own anatomies, thereby keeping intersex secret within families. Such secrecy upholds the perceived social prohibition on intersex, but, as we will see, it damages each child's opportunity to cultivate a mind of their own. To explain how this happens, it is helpful to leverage a theory of child development that, unlike Bowlby's behaviorally oriented account, places the unconscious center stage. Psychoanalysis provides such a theory. For analysts including Torok and Nicolas Abraham, with whom Torok frequently collaborated, human psychological life originates in infantile union with the mother, preceding individuality. That is to say, in early infancy we all exist in a state of "dual unity" between mother and child.[51] Rather than being a period of absolute fusion, dual unity is best understood as an intimate dyad.[52] Its dyadic nature is important because it means that from the start a child "has no conscious or unconscious other than that of his mother," in

Abraham's words.[53] In this sense, though the child is always distinct from the mother, the close dependency on her body and gestures means that the child experiences a foundational "direct empathy" with the mother's mental life, unmediated by representational thought.[54] Out of such unity comes what Abraham, Torok, and other psychoanalytic thinkers call *individuation*—a gradual psychological differentiation into individuality. The child is reliant on the mother throughout development both to sustain union and to allow individuation.[55] In the context of the present chapter, this account challenges the presumption that the minds of parents and children are radically dissimilar. It also implies that instead of focusing on how the child represents the parents (in working models of attachment figures) or on how the child becomes like them (in identifying with certain behaviors), our discussion should shift to examine how the child becomes separate from them. Separate but not radically dissimilar: this is a matter of how the child's individuality unfolds through the relationship between mother and child.

Given the child's reliance on the mother, the unique particulars of her mental life are very significant because they determine the manner in which the child emerges as an individual. From the beginning of the child's life, the mother's words are bound by her specific history of unconscious repressions. Writing on the distinction between the conscious and the unconscious, Sigmund Freud theorized that a "conscious presentation comprises the presentation of the thing plus the presentation of the word belonging to it," whereas an "unconscious presentation is the presentation of the thing alone." By this theory, the capacity to apprehend "the thing alone" without "the word belonging to it" makes repression possible because it means that knowledge can be unstated or expressed indirectly by different words.[56] So the fact that all mothers possess an unconscious means that there is a degree of opacity in what any mother says. During the process of individuation, the child starts to adopt the words of the mother, reusing them to "designate objective events," as Abraham puts it—turning the words "away from the mother's person" and toward "events unencumbered by the mother's unconscious."[57] This act separates the child's conscious and unconscious from those of the mother, earning the child a mental life of their own. However, at the same time the child's individuality remains contingent on "the singular circumstances and psychic traumas of the mother's life," as Rashkin notes in a commentary on Abraham and Torok's ideas.[58] Because the child's mental life is the psychic pattern formed by detaching the mother's words from her person, and because those words are bound by the unique contents of the mother's unconscious, the resulting pattern retains the outline of its origin beyond the child. To phrase this another way, what we think of as the psychology of the child is the boundary etched by division from the "singular circumstances and psychic traumas" of the previous generation. This boundary belongs to the child, but it is also the silhouette of someone else's history.

Successful individuation is therefore dependent on the extent to which a mother can allow her child to uncouple her words from her unconscious. Not all mothers are able to do this. In the event that a mother's words are motivated by what Torok calls "unspoken fears," the child is blocked from detaching her words fully from her person.[59] The words remain encumbered by the mother's repressed knowledge, and, as a consequence, the process of individuation fails to unfasten the child from the mental life of the mother. In such a scenario, the child acquires from the mother "an unknown, unrecognized knowledge," as Abraham and Torok describe it—knowledge that the mother fears to disclose, which continues to freight her words even as they are taken up by her child.[60] Considered in relation to intersex, this scenario suggests that the repressed awareness of the child's atypical anatomy does not remain with the mother alone. This point is demonstrated vividly by the recollection of one former patient, whose intersex characteristics and surgery were undisclosed during childhood. He recounts that "[as a child] I was never allowed to venture further than the sound of Mums [*sic*] voice," adding, "I never knew why," and "I just sort of thought I must have done something really bad."[61] Here, the process of individuation was contorted around an unspoken fear. The mother's demand that the child stay within the range of her voice meant that her words stayed tethered to her person. There was a transmission between the generations, even in the absence of disclosure—an inherited knowledge ("something really bad") that the child could not consciously discern ("I never knew why"). In this fashion, the existence of intersex was neither withheld from the child nor made conscious. Instead, it was passed to the child in an "unknown, unrecognized" form, as Abraham and Torok suggest. Therefore, I argue, contrary to medical traditionalists, that the child *does* have an unconscious. Moreover, there is something inside it that was repressed by the mother, not by the child.

My argument is that children inherit the repression of intersex directly, without being conscious of having had an intersex anatomy. Abraham and Torok give a remarkable name to such a "formation of the unconscious that has never been conscious": They call it "the phantom."[62] Whereas unconscious material is usually defined by its repression from thoughts that were conscious at first, here the repressed material has never been conscious for the child in whose unconscious it resides. Described by Torok as "alien to the subject who harbors it," the phantom personifies the mental presence of something repressed by somebody else.[63] Just as a ghost might traverse the walls of a family house, the phantom in Abraham and Torok's theory traverses the boundaries between family members. Psychoanalytic theorists often associate phantomic haunting with parental silence, but I take a different position, agreeing with Rashkin that to be haunted is to witness "cryptic language and behavior" by one's parents.[64] That is, a child haunted by a phantom has an impression that the parents are concealing something, without understanding the nature of it. In Freud's terms, cryptic parental conduct cleaves "the presentation of the thing" from "the word belonging to it," employing language in obscure and ominous ways. Hence, there was not silence for the former patient who recalled a childhood sense of "something really bad," but rather the sound of his mother's voice. The mother's enigmatic insistence that he should stay close enough to hear her words hinted that something would go wrong if the child were to leave the family and enter the world. I interpret her demand as a coded reference to the prohibition on intersex, which parents ascribe to the world of other people. By following his mother's cryptic instruction to stay close, the child was drawn into maintaining the secret of his genital atypicality without ever knowing that his anatomy was transgressive. In this manner, cryptic conduct by parents leads to intersex being repressed across the generations.

I argue further that the repression inherited by children is, in fact, the very amnesia relied on by clinicians when scheduling surgeries. This original argument reverses the traditional medical view that it is fine for parents to withhold information about intersex because young children are blissfully amnesic. I am claiming the opposite—that young children are amnesic *because* parents repress the knowledge of intersex. Specifically, the cryptic parental speech that arises from their unspoken fears impedes the child's ability to remember experiences. This argument is substantiated by multiple studies in developmental psychology showing that children's capacity to remember events depends on the extent to which their experiences are "linguistically scaffolded" by adults at the time of occurrence. If parents narrate events in an elaborative style, children find it easier to recall the events later. If parents provide no narrative but use language for categorization instead, then recollection is harder for children.[65] So when parents regard their child's genital ambiguity as having "been repaired, and that's it," they talk in ways that actively prevent memory formation: they fail to provide the linguistic scaffold that would enable their child to remember what has happened. Likewise, when parents address their child after genital surgery as a girl or boy, they are using language to categorize, failing to elaborate a narrative that would allow the child to recall experiences prior to surgery. Some parents start categorizing even before surgery has happened: as one mother recounted, once masculinizing surgery was planned, "I went to extremes where I wouldn't buy anything but blue or white, got to be blue."[66] Going to extremes of gendered categorization in this way is done simultaneously to repress one's own knowledge of intersex and to stop one's child from remembering it. So whereas traditionalists presume that children are amnesic because they have no unconscious in which to repress anything, I am proposing that the phenomenon commonly called "childhood amnesia" is really the inherited repression of intersex. Such amnesia keeps intersex secret by making it unspeakable.

I opened this chapter with the question of authenticity. The effect of amnesia is inauthenticity. The psychology of the child that takes shape in a family where intersex is repressed lacks autobiographical coherence; the parents' unyieldingly cryptic speech and behavior cause the child to be unable to retain parts of their autobiography. The deliberate failure by parents to elaborate a narrative of shared events, especially the child's early life with intersex characteristics, leads their child to acquire an inauthentic personal history. Whereas successful individuation would result in the child gaining the ability to use language to "designate objective events," in Abraham's phrasing, the inheritance of parental repression means that the child cannot tell the truth about their own life. Instead, the child's autobiography becomes what Torok has called a "story of fear," distorted by the missing knowledge that parents are afraid to disclose.[67] On this point, the behavioral analysis of attachment converges with the psychoanalytic theory of individuation. Research has found that when children and parents form attachments in an avoidant style, their conversations tend to be less elaborative and interactive. Accordingly, avoidant attachments are associated with children having poorer long-term memories.[68] So when parents say that their genitally atypical child cannot be "accepted for who she is" or cannot "decide for his self" regarding medical treatment, they are doing something more than invoking a perceived social prohibition on living life with an intersex anatomy. I think these parents are also describing the malign consequences of the amnesia that they have caused. Being accepted as oneself and deciding for oneself are impossible in the absence of autobiographical coherence. As Rashkin explains, the phantomic presence of repressed knowledge "blocks the child from living life as her or his own."[69] The argument I have made in this chapter shows that our attachments to others mean that personhood can never be simplistically authentic. Nonetheless, what we inherit through those relationships determines the extent to which our inner lives are haunted by the fears of others.

4

WHAT CAN QUEER THEORY DO
FOR INTERSEX?

To queer and nonqueer folk alike, the visceral immediacy of the sexual touch might appear to be self-evident; contact between a lover's body and one's own is typically coincident with the mutual sensation of such contact. But when the nerves in one's genitalia have been damaged by surgery for intersex, touching is sundered from feeling. Hence, the apparently real-time nature of sexual experience—in which, as the cultural critic Sarah Chinn claims in an essay about queer touching, "our bodies feel and are felt outside solely visual perception"—turns into the static voyeurism of pornography. Touching happens, but it is seen rather than sensed, and in Chinn's opinion vision "is virtually useless when it comes to figuring out and describing the experience of sexual pleasure."[1] The result is isolating and disorienting, as I recounted in chapter 1. It also presents a limit case for queer theory as a school of thought and cultural practice that has attended so prominently to the felt experience of sex acts, as Chinn's comments indicate. Given queer theory's own emphasis on "figuring out and describing the experience of sexual pleasure," one might ask whether there is anything for queer theory to figure out about the postsurgical intersex body. Simply put, when genitalia are damaged after surgery, can queer theory do anything for intersex?

To place this question in context, consider a letter to the influential *Journal of Urology* in 1996, in which the founder of ISNA, Cheryl Chase, described the many sensory problems reported by members of this intersex patient-advocacy group. It was a key early example of intersex patients talking in their own words in a major medical journal, and it coincided with queer theory's rise to academic prominence in the humanities during the 1990s. Chase's letter recounted that several group members experienced either diminished or extinguished genital sensation following surgery. One member whose clitoris was reduced in childhood found orgasm "so difficult to reach and so rarely attained" that she regarded her "sexual function as being destroyed." Disturbingly, another member felt "intense genital pain" following sexual stimulation.[2] Some years later, a study by a London-based medical team evaluated clitoral sensation in six intersex women whose clitorises had been surgically reduced. The study was innovative because it used not merely a sexual satisfaction questionnaire but also electronic devices to measure clitoral sensitivity to temperature and vibration. These devices provided gradually increasing stimuli until participants pressed a button to register sensation. It was the first time that such "objective sensory testing" had been performed on individuals with a history of genital surgery.[3] It was also an opportunity to learn whether Chase's letter was representative.

The results were chilling. In the electronic testing, postsurgical clitoral sensation in the six women was found to be "profoundly abnormal." All had atypical results for the sensation of cold, and five participants had abnormal results for sensations of warmth and vibration. In response to the questionnaire, four women said they had problems achieving orgasm. Worryingly, this atypicality was not just the legacy of outdated surgical techniques: the authors of the study cautioned that "there is currently no justification for the optimism that modern surgical techniques are better for preserving clitoral sensation than previous operations."[4] The caution was an implicit rejoinder to the criticism by earlier clinicians that the individuals discussed in Chase's letter had not benefited from surgical advances made since the mid-1970s.[5] Even if scholars outside medicine might query the London team's claim that a phenomenon as culturally contingent as sexual response can undergo "objective" testing, I think their methodology is still useful in making their study authoritative to other doctors as well as in substantiating the testimonies in Chase's letter.

Might queer theory be useful, too? In this chapter, I want to evaluate whether a critique of these sorts of surgical effects is possible from a queer theoretical perspective on the body. I will make four main claims, beginning with my reservations about queer discourses of pleasure and shame. My first claim will be that the postsurgical body cannot be accommodated by a queer discourse in which sexual pleasure is a form of hedonistic activism. In other words, a queer response to the problems of intersex surgery cannot be simply the advocacy of more and better sex because that is precisely what intersex surgery impedes. My second claim will be that a queer discourse of shame enables a more thoughtful engagement with the surgical creation of atypically sensate bodies, reminding us that such bodies obdurately remember the shameful touch of surgery no matter how desperately we may wish to sweep away its effects. Nevertheless, I do not plan to suggest that critics need simply choose to theorize intersex in terms of either pleasure or shame. There is really no such opposition. That being so, my third claim will be that shame and pleasure are interlinked queer sensations, which together are exemplified by the scintillating caress of the queer touch. Yet queer theory's assumption of a tactile basis to cultural critique flounders when confronted with the desensitized intersex body. In the light of this stalled encounter, my fourth and final claim will be that if queer theory is figured instead as a kind of reaching—but not necessarily touching—then it can better explain the complex aftereffects of genital surgery. Reaching is queerer than touching, for it is a recognition that desire can surpass the limits of the body.

QUEER PLEASURES

On the face of it, queer theory makes possible a critique of diminished sexual pleasure following intersex surgery. This is because queer theory, together with related strands of feminism, is the critical discourse with the most to say about the cultural significance and experience of human sexual pleasure: It is a "vision of social production that engages the libidinal," in Lee Edelman's words.[6] Unlike the emphasis on gender differences in much Western feminist thought and specifically in so-called antisex feminism on sexual pleasure as a ruse of gender oppression, queer theory has taken the sexual realm and its pleasures as central objects of study.[7] A groundbreaking expression of this approach came in 1979 with an article by Patrick Califia in the *Advocate*. Reflecting on Califia's experience of sadomasochistic sex in the San Francisco lesbian community, the article drew a contrast between the "pleasure" of sadomasochism and the subjugation of "real slavery or exploitation." This contrast, which might seem quite obvious to readers now, was provocative at the time because it suggested that sex acts could at once imitate and subvert social structures. Significantly, Califia described sadomasochism's pleasures as "ephemeral," unlike "economic control or forced reproduction." The opposition here was not only between real and simulated subjugation but also between the felt immediacy of sexual activities and the historical weight of sexuality's institutional formations. In this way, sadomasochism could be "time-consuming and absorbing," in Califia's words, paradoxically because its pleasures were transitory—a series of present moments that viscerally enveloped participants.[8] By equating sadomasochism with a unique temporality of pleasure, Califia was able to articulate a position that was neither heterosexual nor antisex. During the 1980s and 1990s, such countercultural possibilities of sexual pleasure would become a central issue for sex-positive feminism and, in turn, queer theory.

The leading theme of Califia's account—sexual pleasure as converse to social structures—will ripple across my present chapter. It has profoundly shaped the interface between queer theory and intersex. An important axiom for queer theorists has been that sex acts can be pleasurable even if or perhaps because they occur outside mainstream norms. This is demonstrated by Califia's contrast between subcultural sadomasochism and the joyless institutionalization of "forced reproduction." Just as a queer discourse of pleasure prioritizes the felt experience of sexual activities, so too have many critics of intersex medicine emphasized the importance of sexual function over norms of genital appearance. For example, in an anthology of writings on queer body image, Chase eschews the cultural use of "infant genitals . . . for discriminating male from female infants" on the grounds that "*my* genitals are for *my* pleasure."[9] Indeed, several intersex activists and scholars have called intersex bodies "queer" in their deviation from expected forms of embodiment.[10] Queer theory and intersex activism converge on the belief that such deviation is not an obstacle to sexual pleasure. Both discourses foreground bodies and communities for whom sexuality functions without adherence to mainstream norms. Queer attention to pleasure is therefore useful in critiquing the normalizing use of genital surgery.

Given that normalcy is not a prerequisite for pleasure, it follows that medical attempts to normalize intersex anatomies have never been primarily about ensuring the capability for pleasure but rather about the capability to conform. This is especially apparent on occasions when clinicians have evaluated vaginal surgery in terms of whether "adequate intercourse," defined crudely as "successful vaginal penetration," is possible postoperatively, and when they have assessed long-term surgical outcomes by whether patients have entered into heterosexual marriages.[11] From a queer perspective, the idea that one might create heterosexual adults by cutting their genitals in childhood severely understates the importance of pleasure to sex and assumes that everyone wants to grow up straight. Although more recent medical guidelines stipulate that "sexual orientation should not be considered as a marker of favorable outcome" of intersex medical management, psychological research into the behaviors of individuals with intersex anatomies is still riddled with stereotypes in which sexual preferences, gender, and sex differences are rigidly aligned. For instance, when such norms are the baseline for what researchers expect to see, the fact that some women with intersex characteristics are nonheterosexual and interested in "rough sports and motor vehicles" stands out, preposterously, as a research finding.[12]

When it comes to contesting sexual and gender norms like these, queer theory has diverged from many Western feminists' endeavor to foster greater parity between existing gender categories. Queer theorists have instead critiqued gender itself for

the perceived limitations that it places on sex acts and sexuality—
arguing that gender categories should be "fucked" (blended,
dissolved, crossed, and so on), as Stephen Whittle puts it suc-
cinctly, instead of defined more equitably between women
and men.[13] Queer theorists have applied similar skepticism to
socially conservative tendencies within sexual communities of all
kinds. This means rejecting the idea that gay, lesbian, and
straight folks have fundamentally common interests in long-term
monogamy, childrearing, and homemaking. For example, Douglas Crimp has eschewed the perceived institutionalism of gay
marriage in favor of the "life-affirming and pleasure-filled
world" of homosexual subculture.[14] More than a critique of gender identity, then, queer theory has enabled a critique of sexual
identity as an essentially conservative concept, too. From this
angle, to identify as gay, lesbian, straight, and so on is conservative because it ties sex acts to a presumed core of personality. It
thereby restricts the meaning of such acts to expressions of the
identity of the person performing the acts. Within queer theory
and communities, sex acts can signify pleasure without reference
to identity. Such resignification even encompasses acts commonly considered heterosexual, for, as Califia has argued, "a
belief in sex differences and a dependence on them for sexual
pleasure is the most common perversion."[15] This is to suggest
that heterosexual sex is not motivated by heterosexual identity
after all; it is merely one kink among many, pursued for pleasure while overlaid by privilege. Queer theory hereby throws into
relief the privilege that accrues to the inhabitants of certain identities regardless of the kinds of sex they may have.

The tensions between privileged and marginalized sexual
identities were heightened during the AIDS crisis of the 1980s.
The epidemic was a life-and-death clash over who had the power
to determine what sex acts signified—from newspaper headlines

that "straight sex cannot give you AIDS" to comments by medics that gay men were like infectious mosquitoes going "from anus to anus."[16] For campaign groups such as the AIDS Coalition to Unleash Power (ACT UP), it was silence, not gay sex, that meant death. During this time, the work of the social critic and cultural historian Michel Foucault was an inspiration for gay and lesbian activists.[17] Translated into English at the end of the 1970s, *The Will to Knowledge*, the first volume of Foucault's *History of Sexuality*, offered a sweeping account of sex and power. As David Halperin has noted in a study of Foucault's influence, the public response to AIDS in the United States during the 1980s perfectly illustrated "the mutual imbrication of power and knowledge" concerning sex that Foucault's book foreshadowed— for example, the "endless relays between expert discourse and institutional authority" that marginalized affected communities. Consequently, AIDS activism multiplied "the sites of political contestation" to encompass "the public and the private administration of the body and its pleasures." This strategy was Foucauldian because like *The Will to Knowledge* it recognized the body as irreducibly political.[18] In the book, Foucault asserted that sexuality is "organized by power in its grip on bodies and their materiality, their forces, energies, sensations, and pleasures" and recommended that power's grasp should be resisted by "bodies and pleasures."[19] Foucault argued, in other words, for bodily pleasure as a way to challenge power.

Within queer theory, there have emerged two distinct views on the relation between bodies and pleasures. According to one view, pleasure is obtained exclusively or most effectively through use of the genitalia. Hence, for activist groups such as Queer Nation, genitalia are "not just organs of erotic thanksgiving, but weapons of pleasure against their own oppression," in the words of Lauren Berlant and Elizabeth Freeman.[20] What makes such genital terrorism queer is the combination of genitalia in a given sex act; queer sex for that reason can terrify and transform heterosexual culture at the same time as it feels good. This is what Tim Dean has described as queer theory's "insistence on the specificity of genital contact as the basis for all political work."[21] In the other view of the relation between bodies and pleasures, queer pleasure is characterized by a focus not on genitalia but on the body as a whole. For example, according to Mark Blasius, homosexual relations become queer when they use "every part of the body as a sexual instrument in order to achieve the greatest intensification of pleasure possible." The result is what Halperin calls "a multiplication of the sites of political contestation" all over the body.[22] From this distinctly Foucauldian standpoint, queer sex can effect cultural change through its stylized attention to reciprocal pleasure, quite aside from its participants' genital morphologies.[23] The latter view is notable also for the continuity that it signals between queer theory and some strands of feminism that seek to make heterosexual relations "nongenitally organized."[24] For writers such as Califia, sadomasochism is paradigmatic of such relations.

In both views, the valorization of pleasure in queer subcultures can be a source of pride. But I think the capacity of the postsurgical intersex body to participate in such subcultures is unclear. Chase, left anorgasmic after genital surgery, has criticized "sex radicals and activists" whose reactions to the nerve damage caused by surgery have ranged from suggesting that one can simply "learn how to orgasm" after clitorectomy to insisting that Chase is actually experiencing "full-body orgasms" but just does not know it.[25] These reactions reflect both queer views on the relation between bodies and pleasures, with the former response centering on the prospect of recovering genital pleasure ("learn how to orgasm") and the latter investing in nongenital pleasure ("full-body orgasms"). But as Chase has commented, both reactions are highly patronizing. I argue that when queer theory focuses on pleasure alone, whether exclusively genital or diffusely full-body, it risks characterizing postsurgical intersex bodies as impoverished because of their diminished capacity for sexual pleasure. In like manner, queer critiques of intersex medicine that are advanced on the grounds that presurgical bodies are queer in their physical divergence from norms may cast postsurgical bodies as less queer (or not queer whatsoever) because of the destruction of genital ambiguity. In summary, bodies damaged by intersex medicine have no easy home within queer communities for whom the experience of pleasure outside mainstream norms is foundational. So it is time to consider whether a different strand of thought within queer theory can make space for intersex.

SHAME AND SHATTERING

How we conceive of sexual pleasure determines how we conceive of desensitizing genital surgery as injurious. Although the queer accounts of pleasure that I discussed in the preceding section can mobilize a critique of surgery on the grounds that the loss of sexual pleasure is bad, such criticism depends on the conception of sexual pleasure as something that can be lost. Now if sex is purely pleasurable, and pleasure is the opposite of no pleasure, then it is indeed possible to lose the capacity for and hence the experience of sexual pleasure. However, if sex is something more or other than pleasurable, then pleasure's presence and absence are not necessarily opposed. Accordingly, the idea of lost sexual pleasure is not straightforward. While some queer theory, in line with much gay pride discourse, has measured the effects of homophobia by the extent to which such prejudice limits subcultural sexual pleasures, other queer theorizations of sex have been more equivocal. Specifically, they have queried the Foucauldian conception of sex as a matter of bodies and pleasures, for, as Sally Munt argues, however "strategically essential" pride in sexual dissidence may be, "the presence of shame has been repressed in the discourse of homosexual rights in an unhelpful way, and in order to gain greater agency, we must learn to revisit its ambivalent effects."[26] In light of Munt's claim, I want to evaluate what queer attention to shame, rather than to pleasure, might do for intersex.

Within queer theory, the most well-known account of sex—and not merely queer sex—as an experience more ambivalent than pleasurable was given by the cultural theorist Leo Bersani in the essay "Is the Rectum a Grave?" in 1987. The essay's incendiary title reflects the fact that Bersani was writing in reaction to the AIDS crisis. Whereas Halperin and others propounded a Foucauldian turn to bodies and pleasures as a means to resist the structures of power and knowledge that conflated homosexuality with social collapse and death, Bersani's response to the same epidemic was to query whether homosexuality is, after all, in some way antithetical to the social realm. In essence, this argument takes queer resistance against socially conservative visions of sexual identity and community to the most drastic conclusion. The big secret about all sex, Bersani advances, is that "most people don't like it"—despite the fact that many people think about sex a lot and want to have plenty of it. Bersani's point is that sex is not as pleasurable as it might seem to us while we fantasize about it. When we actually have sex, Bersani claims, we are no longer self-contained subjects enjoying an easily quantifiable experience of pleasure that we have envisioned beforehand. Quite the reverse: For Bersani, sex is an experience of radical dissolution that is best described as "self-shattering."[27] The dissolution of the self through sex undoes, in turn, the bonds that hold couples and communities together.[28] The desire for sex is therefore "socially dysfunctional," says Bersani, irrespective of whether it entails vanilla heterosexual intercourse or the genital terrorism of groups such as Queer Nation. Regardless of the number of participants, their sexual preferences, or their political slant, sex is a profoundly atomizing affair. Though the reach of this argument is universal, Bersani enlists gay sex as a central exhibit. In Bersani's account, the passive "suicidal ecstasy" of the gay bottom exemplifies self-shattering and is a mascot for the general theory of sex as nonrelational.[29] This idea has subsequently become known as the "antisocial thesis" in queer theory.[30]

The antisocial account of sex puts in question the apparently self-evident problem of desensitizing genital surgery. If sex is not pleasurable anyway, then the diminution or loss of sexual pleasure is a misnomer or perhaps a tautology. It is a misnomer if something other than pleasure is lost to postsurgical sex. It is a tautology if a loss of pleasure characterizes sex in general. A way to resolve this conundrum would be to say that self-shattering is really just another name for pleasure, which is what Bersani argues elsewhere about the apparent pain of masochism.[31] But rather than try to sanitize such shattering by defending it as "pleasurable debasement," the antisocial thesis in queer theory has developed into a complex discourse about negativity, futurity, and—most significantly for my argument here—shame.[32] In short, this discourse holds that the antisocial character of sex—debasing, disintegrating, demeaning—makes sex shameful. Queer subcultures have a distinctive relationship to such shame, some critics have argued; if sex for both queers and nonqueers is a kind of shattering, then what distinguishes queer subcultures is not the performance of certain sex acts (genital terrorism, whole-body sadomasochism, or anything else) but a particular attitude toward the antisocial experience of sex. According to the cultural critic Michael Warner, in queer subcultures "one doesn't pretend to be *above* the indignity of sex" because "we're all in it together."[33] In this way, says Bersani, an "acknowledgement of all that is most abject and least reputable in oneself"—namely, the atomizing evacuation Bersani describes—perversely enables "the special kind of sociability that holds queer culture together."[34] That is to say, queer subcultures are characterized by the recognition that sex is antisocial.

Nonetheless, if sex is really as shamefully antisocial as Bersani describes, we have to wonder why people have sex at all. This is a serious point. Even though Bersani aims to "desexualize the erotic" by casting it as antisocial, Bersani's account remains resolutely sexualized in its valorization of gay anal penetration as the exemplary "intensification or . . . mode of revelation of an always-already shattering self," as Kathryn Bond Stockton comments.[35] As a consequence, there is a circularity in Bersani's argument. Bersani explains, through reference to sex, that "most people don't like sex" because they have had it but disliked the way in which it shattered them. This does not account for those people who have not had sex, cannot have it, or do not want to have it in the first place. Yet I think the latter people may be no less queer. A critique of queer theory by Heather Love is useful on this point. Love has argued that "queer desire is often figured as . . . excessive, dissonant desire. But it would also make sense to understand queerness as an absence of or aversion to sex."[36] Both types of queerness presented by Love are possible on the basis of the antisocial thesis, but much queer theory has alighted on the first—queerness as an excessive embrace of shameful shattering—while failing to investigate the second, queerness as a rejection of or withdrawal from sex.

The absence of sex, as Love admits dryly, is "not very sexy," and for that reason it received little critical attention during the early years of queer theory.[37] But if queer theory is to do anything for intersex, it needs to theorize the ways in which postsurgical bodies may be asexual and even downright unsexy to some people—including sometimes those of us who dwell in such bodies. The shattering experience of sex might be shameful—the antisocial thesis teaches us that much—but not having sex or having sex without shattering can be shameful, too. In queer discourse, the figure of the stone butch is sometimes presented as the personification of the absence of or the aversion to sex described by Love. Traditionally, a stone butch makes love to a femme partner but refuses to be touched in return. Being stone can therefore seem like a disconnection from erotic experience—the polar opposite of the gay bottom in Bersani's account. As such, the figure of the stone butch potentially marks a space for intersex within queer theory. Indeed, in a seminal essay on stone experience and cultural representation, Jack Halberstam has made an argument similar to Chase's complaint that one cannot just learn how to orgasm after a clitorectomy. Contesting the depiction of stoneness as "a wall that has been built up and could come down with the right femme," Halberstam argues that being stone is not an aversion that might be solved by having more sex.[38]

In fact, despite the stone-butch body's "impenetrability," Halberstam suggests that it remains "open to rubbing or friction." To be stone, then, is not a one-way withdrawal from eroticism but "a courageous and imaginative way of dealing with the contradictory demands and impulses of being a butch in a woman's body."[39] Because of this, I believe there are two critical reasons why the stone butch is not truly a model for what queer theory might do for intersex. First, stone butch is an identity, whereas intersex is an anatomy; I do not think there are intersex people in the same sense that there are (for example) lesbian people.[40] Some individuals do identify as *intersex* or *intersexual*, of course, and I use the word *intersex* throughout this book. But I still do not hold that it is comparable to *lesbian* or *stone butch* because to say that *intersex* names an identity specific to a certain anatomy would be to imply that the identities with which intersex is compared are grounded in anatomy, too. Taken to the extreme, this can imply that everyone under the LGBTQI+ umbrella has a biologically based identity.[41] Tying identity to anatomy would not be queer at all, and stone butches show already that one's body does not dictate one's identity—hence, the "contradictory demands and impulses" that can arise, as Halberstam says. The second reason why stone butch and intersex are unalike returns us to the issue of sensation with which I opened this chapter. Because the queerness of the stone butch lies not in sexual closure but in the performance and reception of certain kinds of touching, "butch untouchability multiplies the possibilities of touch," as one commentator on Halberstam's work has noted.[42] In this regard, the stone-butch body is still a tactile body. It is therefore vital to examine whether there is a similar place for the postsurgical intersex body in the relationship between queerness, tactility, and touch.

MINORITY SENSATIONS

Writing on touch is often an occasion to comment on the human condition. In a major book on the topic, the anthropologist Ashley Montagu once advised gravely that "inadequate tactile experience will result in . . . inability to relate to others in many fundamental human ways."[43] In this fashion, touching has frequently been presented as both figure and ground for interpersonal relations: it at once exemplifies relations and makes them possible. This is because the touch, in Margrit Shildrick's words, is "an undecidable moment of exchange" during which one's "sense of wholeness and self-sufficiency dissolve."[44] Here is shattering not as antisocial but conversely as the basis for sociality. Accordingly, several queer theorists and feminists have celebrated the "conjoining power of touch" as ethically and sexually superior to what Shildrick calls an anesthetic ethic grounded in "separation and division" that some critics have associated with the sense of sight.[45] The idea that queer theory itself is a kind of touch has been formatively elaborated by the scholar Carolyn Dinshaw in an essay titled "Chaucer's Queer Touches/A Queer Touches Chaucer," which I will circle around in this section of the chapter.[46] The essay is about the experience of reading Geoffrey Chaucer's fourteenth-century *Pardoner's Tale* queerly as a twentieth-century critic. The unusual title of Dinshaw's essay sets the tone for its argument. A moment of undecidable exchange is suggested by the substitution of an ambivalent slash for the conventional academic colon that would hierarchize title and subtitle. What is more, conjoining is expressed by the grammatical chiasmus of "Chaucer's Queer Touches" and "A Queer Touches Chaucer," which indicates that queer criticism will emerge where author and critic touch.

Dinshaw's nonhierarchical configuration of author and critic points to how touching connotes equality between individuals; neither author nor critic alone can make a text queer. Similarly, Warner has used a spatial metaphor to claim that there is equality in shame because in queer subcultures the indignity of sex is "spread around the room, leaving no one out, and in fact binding them together."[47] Shame here touches individuals and connects them, weblike—without the "separation and division" criticized by Shildrick. And just as there is no "sub" in Dinshaw's title, so too has Califia argued that queer sexual practices focused on touching are mutually respectful and nonhierarchical. During gay sex, writes Califia, "there's good sex, which includes lots of touching, and there's bad sex, which is nonsensual," emphasizing that nonpenetrative touching is more than mere foreplay.[48] I think this accent on touch has a temporal aspect, too, recalling Califia's description of sadomasochism as "time-consuming and absorbing": when touching becomes something more important than a step on the path toward penetrative sex, it takes on a languorous temporality of its own. Consequently, in both queer views on the relationship between bodies and pleasures that I discussed earlier, touching is crucial. Although Blasius's model of sex that engages the entire body does demote the genitalia as the primary location of sexual activity, it simultaneously elevates touching, just like the genital-centered behavior that it is intended to supersede.

Queer attention to touch is certainly an effective counterpoint to the medical project of making genitalia look normal at the cost of desensitization. It lets us argue that desensitization is not an acceptable side effect of normalizing surgery because genitalia are for touching, not for looking at. This provides a different angle of critique from complaints that surgery affects reproductive capability and urinary function. But implicit in this type of critique, whereby a medical concern for appearance is distinguished from a queer concern with touching, is a significant conflation of touch and tactility. Touch and tactility are not the same: the former is an action, whereas the latter is a sense. Hence, a body can touch without tactility, for instance, if one's hands are numb from exposure to cold weather. Likewise, a tactile body is not necessarily a body that is touched, as the figure of the stone butch exemplifies. Then again, some bodies are indeed tactile, touching, and touched all at once. Touching and tactility are different, so my point is that they do not always coincide. Crucially, therefore, the conflation of touch and tactility is what enables a queer critique of intersex surgery as an impairment of touch. This is because surgical desensitization impairs touching only if touching is assumed to entail tactility. Desensitized genitals can still touch and be touched; it is their tactility that surgery damages.

More than arguing for a queer critique of the impairment of tactility, I want to consider here whether queerness itself may be a kind of tactility or sensitivity to impressions. Elizabeth Freeman has called queer history "a structure of *tactile* feeling," and I am interested in whether postsurgical bodies can find a home within such a queer sensorial assembly.[49] The shattering experience described by Bersani demonstrates that queer pleasure and shame are not necessarily opposed, for such pleasure and shame are both "sensations of minority," to borrow a delightful phrase from Berlant.[50] But contrary to Halperin and Bersani alike, I think this is not because either one of these sensations is intrinsically subversive. Rather, it is owed to how their interrelationship is cultivated through participation in queer communities. To phrase this another way, pleasure and shame arise simultaneously within bodies that interact outside mainstream heterosexual spaces. Consider in this connection an account by Berlant and Warner of watching a performance of "erotic vomiting" at a leather bar. Describing the audience's transfixion on the performance, Berlant and Warner comment that "people are moaning softly with admiration, then whistling, stomping, screaming encouragements." In other words, the bodies of both the performers and the audience are affected by the scene. For

Berlant and Warner, this is the production via sex in public of "nonheteronormative bodily contexts." The result is a queer community as the audience presses forward into "a compact and intimate group" of bodies before the performers.[51] I would argue that the whole scene—the leather bar, the surging audience, the performers, and, yes, the vomit, too—comes together to form "a structure of tactile feeling," in Freeman's phrasing. In light of this attention to the embodied sensations of minority, we can understand the Foucauldian emphasis on pleasure and the anti-social emphasis on shame—for surely both are in circulation during the erotic vomiting performance—as intersecting strategies to privilege minority sensations. Such sensations not only signal but also actually constitute a resistant relation to mainstream society. When they materialize together, they have countercultural force.

Cultural change, for Dinshaw, is correspondingly accomplished not through touching alone but through the queer sensation of the touch. Dinshaw states that the "disillusioning force" of a queer character such as Chaucer's Pardoner "shakes with his touch the heterocultural edifice": these sensory metaphors of shaking and force describe not only touching but moreover the tactile impression of being touched. Similarly, Dinshaw asserts that twentieth-century readers of the Pardoner "can feel the shock" of the character's discourse and thereby "appropriate that power for queer use." I suggest that queerness in Dinshaw's argument names the simultaneity of touching and tactility. Because of this simultaneity, queerness for Dinshaw can "provoke perceptual shifts and subsequent corporeal response in those touched." It is through queer sensations, then, that cultural change is accomplished. As Dinshaw explains, "queerness articulates not a determinate thing but a relation to existent structures of power. Despite its positioning on the other side of the law, it is arresting: it makes people stop and look at what they have been taking as natural."[52] It is as if bringing power structures and unstructured lawlessness into relation enables some intermingling between these positions—as though making queerness and heterosexual culture touch could reveal that which seems natural to be a construction after all. For folks who can relate to Shildrick's description of touching as an undecidable exchange in which self-sufficiency dissolves, it is easy to imagine that when queerness and heterosexual culture touch, cultural change will happen. But with genitalia of diminished tactility, the catalytic or shattering potential of touching is far less clear. Dinshaw claims later that the queer touch renders strange "what has passed until now without comment."[53] I agree that queerness can have such an effect, but what passes without comment in Dinshaw's own queer analysis is the simultaneity of touching and tactility.

In summary, queerness as a critical kind of touching requires a tactile surface—whether of an individual subject or a cultural structure—for the registration of its contact. This surface also forms the border between the mainstream and the minority, the site where subcultural sensations are excluded from the social realm even as they collide with it. The conflation of touch and tactility in this model of queerness may evidently stigmatize those individuals whose genitalia are without sensation, marking us as unable "to relate to others" and therefore as less than fully human, as Montagu speculated. But that is not my only dispute with this discourse. Rather, I want to make another move: I want to query the assumption that the body produced by normalizing genital surgery "passes without comment" and so is susceptible to queer denaturalization in the manner described by Dinshaw. If we think of surgery itself as touching,

I suggest that its effects are more ambivalent, so a different kind of critique will be necessary.

TOUCHED BY SURGERY

To understand how genital surgery is a kind of touching, it is necessary to unpack an implicit distinction in accounts of the queer touch. The queer touch, as discussed in the previous section, is implicitly organized around a difference between culture and nature, and therein lies a contradiction. On the one hand, the queer touch is unabashedly cultural in its opposition to naturalized structures: it transmits a denaturalizing constructivist force. On the other hand, the fact that the simultaneity of touching and tactility passes without comment in queer discourse is naturalizing: in this regard, the queer touch itself seems beyond construction. This contradiction does not mean that we should abandon the theorization of queer touching, but it does suggest that we should shift the terms in which the touch is theorized away from the opposition between culture and nature. This move will enable a more interesting critique of genital surgery because such a critique will not depend on reaching a judgment about whether surgery purely naturalizes or denaturalizes intersex genitalia.

I argue that genital surgery for intersex is an example of how bodies touch. It is an embodied encounter between patients and surgeons. The operating room, a space of stylized hygiene, makes possible extraordinarily intimate touches in which normally unseen and inaccessible bodily interiors are touched by other bodies and their technological prostheses.[54] Technology such as the scalpel extends the temporal reach of the surgeon's touch.

The scalpel lends the surgeon's touch a force of which durability is an effect: By having the power to cut the body, the surgeon's touch persists in ways that would be impossible otherwise, changing for life the patient's genitalia. As Sara Ahmed has written of embodiment more generally, "The wound functions as a trace of where the surface of another entity . . . has impressed upon the body."[55] In a medical context, the counterpart of the surgeon's movements is the immobility of the patient's anesthetized body, which in its meaty docility is receptive to the impression of the touch. Such docility is an actively generated aspect of surgery rather than a simple passive state. The patient's induced unconsciousness enables bodily resistance to the force of the scalpel, so that pressure increases until the skin is broken. A conscious patient would retreat from the scalpel, reducing the pressure of its touch upon the body and preventing incisions. After surgery, as the pain of wounds fades, the formation of scars constitutes a visual record of the cutting that anesthesia has cloaked from the patient's sight.

In my opinion, the touch of genital surgery on the body is strikingly similar to Esther Newton's classic account of how drag performers incongruously mix "sex-role referents," such as a masculine tuxedo and feminine earrings. The performers in Newton's study called this "working with (feminine) pieces," a phrase that I think describes what surgeons do when operating on intersex anatomies, although the "pieces" are not sartorial items but body parts, and not only feminine ones are manipulated.[56] The surgeon's touch has the force to detach, move, reshape, and injure such pieces. The ensuing "drag" of surgery may involve manipulating conventionally masculine and feminine genital parts, such as a phallus and labia, or it may take the form of juxtapositions between scarred tissue and undamaged flesh. From a queer standpoint, it would be very tempting to argue that genital surgery is a drag act that performatively produces gender by "dragging on" in the life of the postsurgical subject. In some instances, this may be true. However, I do not think we can assume that genital surgery necessarily has anything to do with gender in the everyday sense. It may simply be stigmatizing, and that is all; gender may be formed by other means.[57] Moreover, even as genital surgery attempts to demarcate certain parts as being clearly masculine or feminine, it fails to do so conclusively—creating, for example, a penis or clitoris that looks about right from a distance but not from up close.

Therefore, this is drag not as disguise or impersonation but as a fragmentary working with pieces whereby the postsurgical body neither remains intersex nor becomes convincingly nonintersex. That body is readable incongruously as both at once, so that one's sexual anatomy seems both glaringly unusual and yet brutally normalized. This is a reason why postsurgical individuals may be fearful of sexual relations.[58] Surgery can leave one unsure as to whether an explanation for one's genital appearance and function needs to be given to sexual partners—and if so, whether such an explanation should presume that partners have already noticed the effects of intersex development, of surgery, or of both. A long way from being genital terrorists, those of us who have had childhood surgery for intersex can sometimes feel terrorized by our own genitalia. As the psychologist Lih-Mei Liao notes, some of us find ourselves during sex "checking what surgeons have done."[59] The deficiency of the distinction between cultural and natural as a framework for understanding genital surgery becomes apparent here: the postsurgical body is neither successfully constructed by surgery into a clearly male or female form, nor is it still naturally intersex. At the same time, depending on who is looking, the body's intersex condition may seem to be an unnatural remnant that has not been adequately naturalized by surgery. So the effect of the surgeon's touch is highly ambivalent in its production of persistently incongruous bodily "pieces"—masculine and feminine, intersex and non-intersex, presurgical and postsurgical.

For these reasons, we might even conclude that genital surgery makes bodies *more* intersex than they started out, as Morgan Holmes brilliantly posits.[60] Certainly, genital surgery can render strange anatomies that might otherwise have passed without comment. For instance, when I was around eleven, in the school locker room (that fabled location on which some surgeons base judgments about the fate of people whose intersexed anatomies do not receive surgery) I was teased *not* because of intersex characteristics that remained after surgery but specifically because of scars *caused* by surgery.[61] The copresence of presurgical and postsurgical times on my body's surface—the pieces of intersex alongside the pieces of surgery—made my intersex condition less notable but my body more strange. This was a "nonheteronormative bodily context," in Berlant and Warner's phrase, if ever there was one. So although surgery is evidently an instrument of heterosexual culture, I would argue that it is nonetheless a queer practice according to Dinshaw's definition. Surgery is an example of what Freeman has named "temporal drag"—the registration of "the co-presence of several historically-specific events" on bodily surfaces.[62] A body that is bound in temporal drag can make spaces that might otherwise be strenuously heterosexual become rather queer, as in transforming a locker room into a place where straight boys comment on the genitals of another boy.

The diminution of genital tactility is another key way in which a historically specific event persists on the body's surface. As Ahmed explains, "It is through the recognition or interpretation of sensations, which are responses to the impressions of objects and others, that bodily surfaces take shape."[63] I think Ahmed is right but tells only half the story: I argue further that the body's very capacity for sensation is shaped by the impressions of objects and others on its surfaces. One such object is the surgeon's scalpel. The point is not simply that we feel touches, but that certain touches, depending on their force and durability, determine what we are able to feel—whether temperature or vibration, as measured in the London study of clitoral sensitivity, or anything at all. In this way, I concur with the transgender theorist Gayle Salamon that "as a perceived and perceiving entity, the body depends on a substratum of history."[64] Surgery's effects show how tactility, far from being simultaneous with touching, always has a constitutive history. A history of surgery forecloses the kinds of touches that a body can feel and drags the genitalia permanently back into the time of anesthetized insensitivity when surgery took place. Genital surgery thereby limits the extent to which the queer touch can reach people with intersex bodies. This is, perversely, an effect of how surgery queers the body.

REACHING OUT

Can queer theory help us reach a future beyond genital surgery? Halberstam has suggested that queer subcultures create "alternative temporalities," freeing their participants from narrative enslavement to the tedium of "birth, marriage, reproduction, and death."[65] There is an affinity here between queerness and intersex because both phenomena can disrupt the heterosexual scripts for birth, marriage, and reproduction. However, to accomplish this disruption, queer subcultures tend to emphasize flexibility in desires, practices, and identifications. This leads to an opposition between flexibility and inflexibility, which in Halberstam's words "ascribes mobility over time to some notion of liberation and casts stubborn identification as a way of being stuck in time, unevolved, not versatile."[66] My concern in this final section of the chapter is with the flexible/inflexible binary itself. The queer touch is emblematic of flexibility because in Dinshaw's formulation it "moves around, is transferable," and can even work "across time."[67] Here I will consider whether the postsurgical body may be more flexible than a queer account might suggest. Yet I will also make an original argument that the flexibility of the postsurgical body should not be the only measure of its future—or, indeed, the measure of only its future.[68]

Even though the postsurgical body of diminished tactility is unquestionably material, it is still constructed, and in a queer reading this may imply a capacity for future change. As I have demonstrated, to say that the intersex body is constructed is to describe its materiality as being contingent on the enduring touch of genital surgery. It is not to imply that the body is unreal, but to tell the history of its realness—and thereby to insist that its realness is worth explaining. Contrary to most commentaries on intersex in the humanities, I offer this account as a caution to queer theorists rather than as a rejoinder to medicine. Queer theory as much as medicine has overlooked the construction of the tactile body, which includes the nurturing of tactility for some bodies as well as the destruction of tactility for others, despite the queer constructivist agenda and its attention to other aspects of the body's cultural formation. Moreover, there is no necessary relation between the revelation of the postsurgical body's construction and its resignification as something else. It may resist such flexibility. So whereas queer theorists often assume that change follows from the revelation of cultural construction, revealing the constructed character of the postsurgical intersex body makes possible no change: the insensate genitalia remain.

In much queer theory, the idea of cultural change is sexualized as the hope for a future in which sex will take place, whether inside or outside the social realm. For example, the activist and writer Amber Hollibaugh once declared that "there is no human hope without the promise of ecstasy."[69] On this point, I think the cultural critic Donald Morton was correct to complain in a heated essay in the mid-1990s that "when queer theorists envision a future, they portray an ever-expanding region of sensuous pleasure, ignoring the historical constraints need places on pleasure." Although I disagree with much of Morton's essay—in particular its simplification of the problems with queer politics to a flimsy opposition between "ludic" postmodernism and materialism—I think Morton was right to critique the assumption that a queer future must be a "sensuous" one.[70] But whereas Morton characterized the historical constraints on queer sensations as matters of material need, in the case of intersex a sensuous future is apparently closed down by the body's history of surgery. In other words, the problem with genital surgery for a queer account of intersex is surgery's foreclosure of the flexibility privileged in queer subcultures and exemplified by touching.

Nevertheless, to align what Salamon calls the body's "sedimented history" with material need versus ludic sensuality would be to give the postsurgical body an unwarranted inevitability.[71] My objection to this alignment is not, for the reasons I explained in the previous section, that it would naturalize the body. Rather, I am concerned that a critique of queer sensations from the point of view of Morton's "historical materialism" would turn that critique into a reiteration of surgery's enduring effects. Put another way, history would come to mean inflexibility. In Morton's attack on queer theory, history (as though this were a singular "systematic development," in Morton's phrase) becomes an explanation for pleasure's limits and thereby imposes a limit of its own on critical analysis: History becomes the boundary beyond which critique cannot pass.[72] Although Morton does not say so, this is because critique itself is a historical formation. So although history may explain why a sensuous future may be problematic, history's force as an explanation cannot be theorized in Morton's critical framework. Similarly, to represent the desensitized intersex body as the historical cause of a future without sex is to fail to imagine that anything other than tactility might organize sex. Therefore, instead of critiquing queer theory in Morton's style by hammering it over the head with historical materialism, we might usefully unravel the opposition between historical inflexibility and queer flexibility.

Desire unravels this opposition, I believe. Consider that a diminution or loss of genital sensation may have nothing to do with desire, which might function independently of tactility. David Reimer, whose alleged sex reassignment from male to female after a circumcision accident in the late 1960s was often cited as proof of surgery's capacity to change gender identity in children with unusual genitalia, once described the persistence of desire following the loss of the penis. "If you lose your arm," Reimer explained to a biographer, "and you're dying of thirst, that stump is still going to move toward that glass of water to try to get it. It's instinct. It's in you."[73] In this comment, Reimer differentiates between desire and history, but for Reimer, unlike for Morton, they are not mutually exclusive. Morton regards desire in queer and postmodern theory as "an autonomous entity outside history," opposed to historically determined need.[74] Desire in Reimer's account, though, is neither wholly inside nor wholly outside history, for it is the experience of the past's failure to determine fully the present. Therefore, although history persists in the present by leaving the postsurgical individual with a "stump," whether literally or metaphorically, the stump may be invested with desire in ways that cannot be anticipated by a historical materialist explanation of how the stump came to be. Said another way, desire arises in the difference between past and present, but it cannot be reduced to an effect of the past on the present. Desire in my analysis is therefore separate from the question of how we might imagine a queer future. It is a matter of how we inhabit the present.

So desire is also distinct from the issue of how we might pursue a queer history as Dinshaw envisages it. At first glance, Reimer's account is akin to Dinshaw's theory of the queer touch: a text such as the *Pardoner's Tale* may activate readerly desires that cannot be explained by the history of the text. These desires arise when text and critic come into contact across time, as Dinshaw says. Yet there is a key difference between Dinshaw and Reimer: The former describes touching; the latter, reaching. Although the reach does not "move around" quite like the touch, it is nevertheless a dynamic "mov[ing] toward," to use Reimer's phrase. Desire in this way cannot be reduced to an embodied affect, for its situation is neither in the presurgical body nor in the postsurgical body. Desire instead names a relation between these bodies for the individual who inhabits the narrative of their succession. Reimer's narrative of reaching interestingly demonstrates both the flexibility of desire and desire's stubbornness—its persistence after genital modification signals desire's adaptability just as much as its intractability. This account of desire thereby confounds the canonical queer binary between flexibility and immobility.

Edelman has argued that queer theory should "remind us that we are inhabited always by states of desire that exceed our capacity to name them."[75] If Edelman is correct, then I think a queer understanding of the postsurgical body need not center upon the genitalia on which surgery operates and that surgery attempts to name as female or male for heterosexual ends. Other types of critique can make those complaints. A queer understanding ought to attend instead to the desires that exceed such naming. Otherwise, queer theory may mirror the medical attempt to normalize bodies as markers of desire by attempting to locate within bodies the countercultural sensations of minority. What queer theory can do for intersex, then, is critique genital surgery without presuming to know in advance what comes after surgery, after desensitization, or even after queer theory—shame or pleasure; naturalization or denaturalization; touching or reaching. I argue that queerness is useful instead for its interrogation of the meaning of the "after," which is the flexibility and inflexibility of history in the present.

5

IN SEARCH OF MEDICAL POWER

I want to open this discussion with two ideas about medical power that circulate widely in critical and activist discourses on intersex medicine. The first is that contemporary medical power over intersex is a distinctively late-modern phenomenon, taking shape in the latter half of the twentieth century and persisting into the twenty-first century.[1] The second is that intersex ought to be released from such power, either entirely or to some degree.[2] So whether critics and activists want merely to lessen the grip of medical power or overthrow it altogether, we all need to know what such power looks like and how it works. In this chapter, therefore, I am going to investigate the form taken by medical power over intersex bodies in late modernity. On the face of it, this ought to be an easy task. A field guide to medical power might say that as intersex bodies are subjected to ever more diagnostic tests, genital surgeries, hormonal interventions, and elaborate clinical surveillance, medicine becomes ever more powerful. Such an account would equate the strength of medical power with the intensity and visibility of medicalization. I would describe that as a linear view of power, in which power seems to function on a sliding scale between, at one extreme, complete dominion over intersex bodies and, at the other extreme, total withdrawal from them. In a linear view like this, power and medicalization operate in lockstep; accordingly, the liberation of intersex bodies from medical power is a matter of their demedicalization. Yet I think power dynamics in late modernity are more slippery than that and not so linear. We oversimplify how power works if we regard medical power as simply proportional to medicalization. We also miss an important opportunity to challenge it. This chapter is going to take up that opportunity by decisively rethinking the power over intersex wielded by medicine in late-modern times.

The reason why power and medicalization do not operate in lockstep is that medical power has a fragile and elusive form, whereby it simultaneously encroaches on intersex bodies and retreats from them in failure. As a result, even though nobody would dispute that intersex is thoroughly medicalized, it is oddly difficult to specify the power that intersex medicine actually wields. When we look for evidence of what medicine achieves with respect to intersex, we find it riddled with gaps—surgeries that do not work, complications and scarring, ambiguous outcomes, and missing data.[3] We see stakeholders on all sides—parents, affected individuals, clinicians, and other specialists—saying how hard it is to make decisions about medical treatments.[4] We find doctors admitting that sometimes no treatment decision can be satisfactory.[5] These well-documented deficiencies seem to be irreconcilable with the dogged persistence of intersex medicine in late modernity. Such irreconcilability underscores why a new interpretation of medical power is urgently required. In what follows, I will argue that the problems with medicine are not incidental to its endurance, but integral to its power. A perennially bungling enterprise, the medical management of intersex places its own authority in doubt by creating bodies that are chronically strange, wounded, and inconclusively sexed. So the issue is not that medicine grants doctors and parents unbridled dominion over intersex bodies but instead that medicine both provokes and constrains them to exercise power through treatment decisions that are irreducibly difficult and even futile. I will show that the intense difficulty of making such decisions creates in doctors and parents a sense of struggle about how to handle intersex. Rather than this inner struggle being a sign that medical power has failed, I shall reveal that it is the most subtle mode of power's operation. It is how power disappears into a private dilemma. At the vanishing point of privacy, medical power escapes public scrutiny and endures precisely because it is so difficult to wield.

THEORIZING MEDICAL POWER

Doctors themselves do not explicitly theorize the power that they hold in relation to intersex bodies, but they have a strong implicit conception of its nature, nonetheless. They conceptualize it as the power to create normality. For example, when they write that the aims of genital surgery are to "correct any structural abnormalities" and make genitalia that are "normal-looking and functioning," doctors claim for themselves the power to normalize intersex bodies.[6] They also recognize that at times this power goes askew. Doctors characterize such lapses as complications—occasions when surgeries do not produce normality but generate "residual problems with sexual and/or urinary function."[7] I suggest that normalization and complications together form a conceptual frame through which doctors perceive and exercise their power. Like any framing device, this frame posits both an interior and an exterior by defining a boundary between them. By establishing such a boundary, the frame separates the successful operation of medical power from its failure. Within the frame, medical interventions appear not to injure the body but to make it normal; outside the frame, certain consequences of the same interventions appear to be side effects that elude the power of medicine.

Yet many intersex critics and activists have rejected this way of framing medical power on the basis that treatment interventions are not a matter of normalization. They have insisted instead that childhood treatments for intersex amount to "state-sanctioned violence" against nonnormative bodies, as the intersex rights advocate Sean Saifa Wall puts it.[8] If such interventions are really acts of violence, then the power that doctors wield when they perform these interventions is not the power to normalize but something crueler and more oppressive. I am going to argue that there are three principal ways in which critics and activists have reframed medical power in our critiques of intersex medicine. The first is to reframe medical power in terms of discipline; the second is to reframe it in terms of regulation; and the third is to reframe it in terms of erasure. The core question addressed by all three alternative frames is: *What does the exercise of medical power mean for intersex bodies, if not normalization?* The frames are not historically sequential or mutually exclusive; all three have circulated in critiques of intersex medicine since the early 1990s. Reframing intersex medicine in these various ways also raises a corresponding question: *What is the form of medical power's failure, if not complications?* In this section of the chapter, I will outline how both power and its failure have been reframed by critics and activists. I will then consider how effective these frames are at challenging the medical conception of power.

Reframed in terms of discipline, the exercise of medical power punishes intersex bodies. An example of a commentator who frames medical power in this way is Anne Fausto-Sterling. As Fausto-Sterling expresses it, "Medical accomplishments can be read not as progress but as a mode of discipline." Reframing medical power as discipline emphasizes that genital surgeries mete out pain and injury to "unruly bodies," in Fausto-Sterling's words, and so constitute a form of rebuke against atypical embodiment.[9] In the discipline frame, the focus of critique turns away from the normal anatomy that surgeons claim to construct toward how the anatomy that already exists is punished by surgical violence. Critics who reframe medical power as discipline therefore see genital surgery as a "coercive violation of bodily integrity" instead of as restorative or benign.[10] The power to discipline intersex bodies is exemplified by the practice of vaginal-construction surgery, which involves pulling open the body using incised flaps of skin.[11] When considered as a disciplinary procedure, such surgery is an act of corporal punishment, not normalization.

Reframed in terms of regulation, the exercise of medical power suppresses intersex bodies. An example of a commentator who frames medical power in this way is Hil Malatino. As Malatino expresses this framing, medical practices are techniques of "intense and intimate corporeal regulation."[12] Reframing medical power as regulation emphasizes that genital surgeries constrain intersex bodies to make them function in ways that go against their nature. Again, the attention in this frame is not on the characteristics that doctors claim to produce; but unlike in the discipline frame, the focus here is on the sense in which medical interventions manipulate existing bodily attributes. The power to regulate is exemplified by the practice of urethral-construction surgery, in which tissue such as the foreskin is cut, moved, and remolded to make a watertight tube on the penis.[13] When considered as a regulatory procedure, such surgery contorts the body into an unnatural state. By performing what Fausto-Sterling calls "the surgical and hormonal suppression of intersexuality," medical power in the regulation frame disfigures atypical bodies in the name of making them appear normal.[14]

Reframed in terms of erasure, the exercise of medical power eradicates intersex bodies. An example of a commentator who frames medical power in this way is Cheryl Chase. Medical practices "erase the evidence from intersexed infants' bodies," Chase writes, to make it seem as if they were never sexually ambiguous.[15] Reframing medical power as erasure emphasizes that genital surgeries diminish intersex bodies by stealing their defining characteristics. The power to erase is exemplified by the practice of clitoral-reduction surgery, which involves destroying a segment of erectile tissue inside an atypically large clitoris, then reattaching the clitoral tip to the stump.[16] In the erasure frame, the elimination of sexual ambiguity is an irreplaceable loss that cannot be mistaken for the establishment of normality; the patient advocate Sherri Groveman, who is Jewish, has described it as a "personal holocaust."[17] The erasure frame also enables a broader critique of the social impact of medicine. By highlighting that "medicalization seeks and maintains invisibility for intersexuality," critics use the erasure frame to reappraise treatments as forms of censorship that make intersex taboo.[18]

Just as the three alternative frames that I have outlined redefine what medical power means, so too do they redefine the meaning of its failure. In the discipline frame, complications signal the body's ability to resist the discipline to which it is subjected. That is to say, surgeries go askew because of "the resistance of the intersexed body," in the words of Myra Hird and Jenz Germon.[19] Reframed in this way, complications are instances of bodily disobedience against power. This point is exemplified by the occurrence of vaginal stenosis, in which a surgically constructed vagina narrows or closes of its own accord.[20] So even though the body that defies discipline does not escape violence, it possesses what critics have named a "resistant biological vitality" to oppose the aspirations of medicine.[21] The discipline frame hereby posits a degree of corporeal agency that exists irrespective of whether patients intentionally reject medical management.[22] Indeed, as we will see, all the critical frames that I am discussing suggest that medical power can fail directly in its encounters with intersex bodies, irrespective of the stance that patients may take toward medical authority or whether they identify as intersex.

In the regulation frame, medical failures are evidence of an excess that escapes being regulated. "The control of the intersexed person's body can never be *total*," Morgan Holmes has insisted, "for the intricacies of both biology and identity are more complex."[23] Reframed in this way, complications are instances of corporeal abundance that evade regulation. This point is exemplified by the occurrence of urethral fistulas, little holes that form in a surgically constructed urethral tube so that it is leaky rather than watertight.[24] Through such postsurgical reactions, the body thwarts the aims of power by erupting into new forms that defy "medical containment," intensifying the body's perceived ambiguity.[25] The regulation frame hereby posits a different flavor of corporeal agency from the discipline frame—one that is less diametrically resistant to power and more floridly anarchic.

In the erasure frame, medical failures are signs of corporeal resilience: despite efforts to eradicate intersex, it endures. "We are who we are," patient support-group member David has protested, "and no amount of surgery and hormones and even conditioning (to the point of brainwashing) can change that."[26] Reframed in this way, complications are proof that the intersex body withstands medical erasure. This point is exemplified by the occurrence of postsurgical clitoral enlargement, when a clitoris that has been reduced in infancy regrows to a larger-than-average size at puberty.[27] In this respect, the erasure frame posits yet another variety of corporeal agency in addition to those within the discipline and regulation frames. Here it is an agency that neither disobeys nor exceeds the exercise of medical power but stubbornly outlasts it.

Through this discussion, we have seen how critics and activists use the three alternative frames of discipline, regulation, and erasure to reappraise both the successes and failures of medical power in terms other than normalization and complications. If power is discipline, then it fails because of bodily resistance; if power is regulation, then it fails because of bodily excess; and if power is erasure, then it fails because of bodily resilience. So these frames are not a set of complaints about the practice of normalization as such; in a deeper sense, they are alternative ways of seeing medical power and its limits. Overall, I think that the contrast between medical and critical frames reflects an inherent ambivalence in the concept of power: it can mean having the power *to do* something, and it can mean holding power *over* someone or something, as social theorists have noted.[28] In the present context, medical power can mean exercising the power to normalize intersex bodies, or it can mean wielding power over them, depending on how such power is framed.[29]

With this contrast in mind, I want to pause for a clarification. Although discipline, regulation, and erasure are readily illustrated by the three varieties of intersex surgery that I mentioned earlier—vaginal construction, urethral construction, and clitoral reduction, respectively—these frames should not be read as synonyms for specific surgical procedures. Rather, they are ways in which intersex treatments of all kinds can be reconsidered as expressions of power over the body.[30] For example, the erasure frame has wider applicability beyond surgeries that remove tissue: the construction of a urethra on a penis can also be framed as the erasure of a penis that has no urethra. Likewise, not merely surgical procedures but also nonsurgical interventions are open to critical reframing—the administration of hormones to affect sex development can be framed as an act of regulation, for instance.[31] In all three critical frames, medical interventions of any type are recast as occasions when power is exercised over intersex bodies—sometimes successfully, sometimes not.

Nonetheless, despite the contrast between medical and critical ways of framing power, I contend that these frames have a fundamentally similar form. I am going to argue that this similarity is problematic. It means that efforts to reframe intersex medicine cannot truly transcend the form of power inherent in medical accounts of normalization and complications. To be specific, the formal element common to both medical and critical frames is the boundary between medical power and its failure. We have seen that in the medical frame this boundary is where the power to normalize the body comes to a halt in the face of complications. We have also seen that in all three critical frames, such complications are interpreted as failures of power over the body—triggered variously by the intersex body's opposition to discipline, escape from regulation, and tenacity to withstand erasure. Therefore, the strategy of reframing medical power has a problem: it replicates medical thought by positing a domain in which power succeeds, demarcating this domain from the defeat of power outside the frame. Said another way, all the critical frames suppose that medical power ends where medical power fails. This is a supposition about the form of power. As a result, each frame can explain only how power produces effects inside the frame. They do not explore how medical power may be implicated in failures that occur outside the frame, such as vaginal stenosis, urethral fistulas, and clitoral regrowth.

I want to take a bolder approach and consider the possibility that we cannot get outside medical power, even when it fails.[32] I realize that it would be possible to argue that the boundary between the success and failure of medical power can be expanded, but then we would maintain the underlying form wherein medical power succeeds on one side of the boundary and fails somewhere beyond it; we would simply broaden what it means for medical power to succeed. To really comprehend the nature of medical power over intersex bodies in late modernity, I think we must reckon with its failures head on. Acknowledging that power fails is just the first step; if we suppose that medical power is limited by its various mishaps, then we still cannot explain its longevity. Given the fact of postsurgical reactions such as stenosis, fistulas, and clitoral regrowth, the puzzle is how medical power persists regardless. We therefore need to make sense of "power in its persistence and instability," to use a phrase from Judith Butler.[33] To start making sense of this puzzle, I would like to turn to the analysis of late-modern power offered by the sociologist and philosopher Zygmunt Bauman in the book *Liquid Modernity* (2000).

We live in "the time of fluid modernity," Bauman's book tells us. Bauman contrasts such fluidity to the preceding era of "heavy capitalism" in which "top-heavy" power fused the accumulation of capital with the organization of physical labor in sites of industrialized production such as factories. During heavy capitalism in the nineteenth century, the exercise of power was visibly located where bodies and capital amassed. But heavy capitalism has been superseded over the course of the twentieth century by today's "dispersed, scattered and deregulated modernity," with corresponding implications for power. Although

Liquid Modernity says little about medicine, I think its central theory hints at the true nature of contemporary medical power over intersex bodies. In the age of liquid modernity, Bauman theorizes, all power is "increasingly mobile, slippery, shifty, evasive and fugitive."[34] This depiction suggests that medical power in the late-modern world cannot be easily framed by anyone because whichever frame is used to conceptualize the boundary between success and failure, power will overflow it. So in the following sections of this chapter, I will not seek to frame medical power at all. Rather, I will explore how medical power is sustained by the creation of bodies for which treatment interventions are neither convincingly successful nor conclusively unsuccessful. As I will suggest in the next section, it is precisely and ironically the indeterminate status of the postsurgical intersex body that causes power relations to proliferate.

POWER AND THE POSTSURGICAL BODY

From my discussion in the previous section, it follows that genital surgery for intersex leaves the body in a state somewhere between the outcomes that doctors call normalization and complications. In other words, as the former patient Tiger Devore has reflected, surgery makes the body "strange-looking."[35] I will argue in this section that the creation of strange bodies not only is an essential function of intersex surgery but also makes its practice characteristic of liquid modernity. Taking up Bauman's thesis that late-modern power is inherently slippery and evasive, I am going to show that the strangeness of the postsurgical body is the mechanism through which medical power circulates and persists in late-modern times. To proceed with my analysis, I want to recognize that there are two sides to the body's role in the operation of medical power. In one sense, the body is the unyielding substance that causes surgical interventions to go askew. In the portrayals of corporeal agency that I outlined in my exploration of framing, we saw that the intersex body is the material through which medical power cannot pass. In this respect, as the sociologists Limor Meoded Danon and Niza Yanay have argued, after surgery the body remains "active and productive, reproducing intersexuality" despite medical efforts to the contrary.[36] But that is not the entire picture. In another sense, the body is the medium through which medical power flows because the performance of surgery cannot be separated from the body. Mobilized by the hands of the surgeon and the instruments of surgery, the anesthetized intersex body is the fleshy vessel through which medical power does its work. In this fashion, genital surgery turns the intersex body against itself, deploying its tissues to dispose of its own intersex characteristics.[37] I think that the two sides of the body's role do not cancel each other out. It has corporeal agency *and* is an agent of medical power too. Therefore, the body holds a divided role as the element in which power simultaneously moves and flounders.

Given the body's divided role and entanglement with medical power, the results of genital surgery are inevitably strange. It is neither the case that normalization fails and the body remains intersex nor that the body is normalized and ceases to be intersex. I think the body instead emerges from its encounter with the scalpel in a peculiar half-damaged, half-restored state. I recounted in chapter 4 how scars do not necessarily replace intersex characteristics or mark the absence of them but coexist with them. Such postsurgical strangeness reflects the uneven passage of medical power through intersex flesh. My interest here lies in how the strange properties of the postsurgical body generate power differentials between individuals who have undergone childhood genital surgery and the people around them. This effect starts from the bewildering experience of finding oneself in a postsurgical body. We have already seen in chapters 2 and 3 that early genital surgery is designed not to be understood by the patient, bypassing integration into the patient's life narrative through the way it is timed and communicated. This means that when early surgery works as intended by doctors and parents, the patient does not remember what the body was like before surgery or even whether surgery took place. But the body remembers. With its uneven textures, visible discontinuities, and leaky gaps, "it is a body that refuses to forget its past," Meoded Danon and Yanay write. In this sense, the postsurgical body recalls a past that the patient never experienced. Even as the body invites interpretation to reconstruct the narrative of events, its strangeness also resists understanding, stirring only "partial knowledge and suspicions."[38] The half-damaged, half-restored body tells a fractured story to the patient. Indeed, the temporal relationship between surgery and bodily marks may be subjectively reversed: for those of us to whom childhood surgeries were never explained, the issue is not that surgery caused scarring but that the belated discovery of scars on one's body triggers a search for their source, so that the effect seems to predate the cause.

Growing up in a postsurgical intersex body is bewildering, then, because the events of early childhood are encoded within one's body in a form that one cannot understand. The fact that one's body *has* a history is self-evident in its ominous scarring and oblique symptoms. Yet the events that compose the body's history are mysterious. We might describe the postsurgical body as the location from which the truth of what happened cannot be seen: from the patient's viewpoint, the reason behind the body's strange characteristics is opaque. There are viewpoints besides this one, though. To other people, the history of the body is clear. It is well known to key individuals around the patient—family members, medical personnel, close family friends, perhaps also babysitters and teachers in whom parents have confided.[39] In fact, the body of a child who receives intersex surgery is an object of scrutiny and discussion far more than it would be without medical intervention and even despite the urgent wish for secrecy, resulting in a foundational lack of privacy for the patient.[40] Therefore, the strangeness of the postsurgical body results in a disparity of knowledge between the patient and other people. The latter know how the body came to be; the former does not. As Michel Foucault often remarked, power actively produces knowledge for those who exercise it at the same time that it blocks or censors knowledge for those who are its target.[41] Owing to this disparity, the patient grows up acutely dependent on knowledge held by others. Although the body after surgery is sufficiently odd to prompt reflections such as *Is that scar where something was taken out of me?* and *Did my genitals always look this way?* the body alone cannot answer these questions. Only other people can. In short, those of us who had intersex surgery in childhood often feel that our anatomy and its treatment are the subject of everyone's knowledge but our own.[42]

I am arguing that the gaps in a patient's knowledge find their complement in the knowledge held by other people who examine and discuss the patient's body. Now I want to go further. I propose that this body serves a social function for others by drawing them together. The context for this provocative claim is that liquid modernity is a time of transient social relationships. During heavy capitalism, public life was already altered by accelerated urbanization, transportation, and information technologies. Around the turn of the twentieth century, the crowded loneliness of cities lit by electric light, the trauma of jolts during

railway travel, and the revolutionary speed of telegraph communication converged to make public life disorienting.[43] As heavy
capitalism then dispersed into liquid modernity, the organization
of labor in sites of industrialized production decreased. As Bauman relates, during the second half of the twentieth century
employment became precarious and shared experiences of work
declined, while urbanization, transportation, and information
technologies accelerated further. The cumulative result, in Bauman's words, was the "falling apart and decomposing of human
bonds, of communities and of partnerships" in the late twentieth
and twenty-first centuries.[44] We already know that swiftly com-
pleted childhood genital surgery and gender assignment emerged
during liquid modernity as the prevalent way to respond to intersex.[45] But I think that such surgery is also a response to the social
experience of liquid modernity. This is because surgery creates
bodies around which people congregate to exchange knowledge:
Social relations are occasioned by the exposure, measurement,
and monitoring of postsurgical intersex bodies. This phenomenon exemplifies what the cultural critic Mark Seltzer has named
"wound culture," a fascination in twentieth-century America
with bodies that are opened and damaged. In wound culture, the
practice of "gathering around the wound" operates as "a version
of collective experience" in lieu of other community bonds.[46] I
argue, therefore, that intersex surgery functions as a specific
solution to a general social problem in liquid modernity, forging
shared experiences by drawing adults around children's bodies
that have been surgically opened.

Where the patient lacks privacy, others gain sociality. When
family members, medical personnel, family friends, and others
congregate to evaluate and discuss the wounds of early childhood
surgery, they share a social experience that is inaccessible to the
patient. The latter's profound dependency on other people for

knowledge about what happened causes a power imbalance between those who gather at the body and the one who inhabits it. There is a relay, then, between the exercise of medical power in the practice of early surgery, the production of knowledge about the resulting body, and the formation of power differentials around the possession of such knowledge. As Foucault has written, "The exercise of power perpetually creates knowledge and, conversely, knowledge constantly induces effects of power."[47] From this analysis, we might conclude that other people know everything that the patient does not—that their power comes from possessing complete information about the postsurgical body. However, I think that such a conclusion would be premature. Although the strangeness of the body after surgery gives people plenty to discuss, it is not because they know everything about it. On the contrary, it is because the results of genital surgery confound definitive interpretation. Clinicians often remark on both the necessity and challenge of assessing the long-term outcomes of intersex surgery—saying, for instance, that the effectiveness of surgical techniques "must await long-term evaluation" even as "evidence-based surgical outcome studies . . . are inherently difficult to perform."[48] There is no consensus on how and when to measure outcomes or even how to quantify the intersex characteristics of the body prior to surgery.[49] Consequently, although those who gather around the body know its surgical history, they remain unsure as to whether the surgery was successful. To put this another way, whereas the patient does not know what happened, other people do not know whether what happened worked.

The account of medical power, knowledge, and the wounded body that I am putting forward here is encapsulated in the practice of follow-up surgeries for intersex. The bodily reactions that I discussed in the previous section—vaginal stenosis,

urethral fistulas, and clitoral regrowth—often move doctors
to undertake follow-up surgeries. These follow-ups can go on
one after another for years. As Meoded Danon notes, "Bodies
may respond to surgeries with unexpected complications and
side effects that lead to repeated surgeries throughout intersex
people's lives."[50] I cautioned earlier that we should not equate
the strength of medical power with the intensity of medicalization. Follow-up surgeries show how medical power overflows
the boundary between success and failure and thus prolongs
medicalization. It is precisely because intersex surgery leaves the
body in a half-damaged, half-restored state that medicalization
continues through follow-ups. In my own personal case, the
unexpected results of an operation at age three led to seven more
surgeries before the age of five. Each follow-up was intended to
remediate the unplanned consequences of the one before, a
promise of normalization that was repeatedly deferred. From the
viewpoint of patients like me who undergo multiple surgeries
early in life, every follow-up increases the obscurity of how one's
anatomy came to be, overlaying new scars on the body. Follow-
up surgeries feel to young patients lacking knowledge of the narrative of events like aftershocks from an unknown origin. For
me, the number of childhood surgeries remained obscure for a
long time. When I read my labyrinthine medical records in
adulthood, I thought there had been six follow-ups, but when I
reread them decades later, I understood that there were seven.
For the people around me, that meant seven occasions to gather
around my postsurgical body, congregating in a shared experience of wound culture as they decided what to do next. Follow-
ups like these demonstrate that when surgeries go askew, not
only medicalization escalates; social bonds intensify, too.

As follow-up surgeries and their effects proliferate, it becomes
increasingly hard for people around the patient to know what

medicalization has accomplished. At once the target, vehicle, and adversary of medical power, the body spurs the pursuit of medicalized solutions to intersex that never arrive. Therefore, although a power imbalance exists between the patient and other people, the power that those people wield as they gather around the postsurgical body is slippery and fragile. The more they exercise their power to normalize the intersex body, the stranger the body gets, and the certainty of their knowledge slips away. Because the knowledge that they possess is unstable, so too is the power that they hold in relation to the patient. Yet in late-modern times there is no conflict between the instability of knowledge and the possession of power. I argue that by generating power relations founded on uncertainty, the surgical practice of making intersex bodies strange is typical of liquid modernity. Bauman posits in *Liquid Modernity* that "the prime technique of power is now escape, slippage, elision and avoidance."[51] This description is borne out by studies of conversations between healthcare professionals and the families of children with intersex characteristics. In one such study, Stefan Timmermans and colleagues observed that "clinical uncertainty and ambivalence" about whether to do childhood surgery enabled medical authority to thrive. In the absence of clear-cut ways to determine the purpose, timing, and effects of early surgery, the conversations that occurred were not demedicalized. Rather, they remained preoccupied with weighing surgical options, preserving the professional power of clinicians, and "leaving a medical framing intact," Timmermans and colleagues found.[52] That is the liquidity of power in action. Whether the number of surgeries is one or many, people around the patient make medicalized decisions because they do not know what to do—and once they make those decisions, they do not know what they have achieved. This power is a slippery and evasive kind, indeed.

In the next section, I will explore how medical power continues to function even when it seems not to exist at all.

SUBJECTS OF STRUGGLE

I have suggested that genital surgery is chosen on behalf of children by adults who are unsure whether such surgery has worked previously or whether it will work in the future. Given my exploration of power in this chapter, it would be easy to condemn the fact that medical decisions about intersex are based on inadequate knowledge—that they are hasty and hubristic. However, that is not the argument I plan to pursue here. In this section, I want to move in a different and original direction by openly recognizing the problem of wielding medical power for those who possess it. Put simply, making irreversible decisions from a place of irreducible uncertainty is really hard. In the words of one group of physicians, "These clinical situations can often be difficult to manage, particularly in those cases where the gender of rearing is uncertain."[53] When attempting to choose treatments and predict outcomes for intersex patients, clinical teams are sharply aware that they lack a "crystal ball."[54] So although medics exert power through the surgical modification of children's intersex bodies, they experience that power very differently—not as a position of control, but as one of upheaval and doubt. "I think we're all in a dilemma about how we continue to practice," conceded an anonymous healthcare professional in an interview with researchers.[55] Comments like this express deeply felt professional anxiety over the medical management of intersex. Some medics hope that involving parents in treatment decisions can defuse the problem. Yet opening decisions to parents raises further challenges: When giving parents advice, clinical teams feel that they do not know what to say.[56] Consequently, parents, too, "are living with massive dilemmas in terms of if they do or don't have treatments," the anonymous interviewee added.[57] Given that decisions about intersex are so intractable, I acknowledge that it might seem simplistic and unfair to criticize those who make them. With no readily available solutions, responding to intersex is certainly "difficult and stressful" for medics and parents alike.[58]

Nevertheless, nothing should be beyond criticism, including the sentiment that intersex medicine is difficult. Though it is true that adults find themselves in a hard position when making poorly informed decisions about children's intersex bodies, that does not mean their position should be exempt from critical scrutiny. On the contrary, it means that critical scrutiny of treatment decisions should include an explanation of the difficulty with which such decisions are made. If we grant that the medicalization of intersex is worth critiquing, but we exclude from critique the sense of difficulty that doctors and parents experience, then we imply that such difficulties are peripheral to medicalization. But I have argued in this chapter that the chronic failure to normalize intersex bodies is a central feature of intersex medicine. Similarly, if we hold that medical power deserves interrogation, but we do not interrogate the dilemmas experienced by doctors and parents, then we imply that those dilemmas arise in the absence of power. But I have suggested that power has no outside, so we should approach the sentiment of difficulty that surrounds intersex medicine with critical skepticism and curiosity—as a phenomenon that may be quietly integral to medicalization as well as characteristic of power. This is the phenomenon of being "in a dilemma about how we continue to practice" while practicing nevertheless. I want therefore to understand how the intractability experienced by doctors and parents can coexist with childhood genital surgery without bringing it to a halt. Put the other way around, I am interested in how the practice of intersex surgery elicits and accommodates discontent and disappointment among the very individuals who choose to do it. As two major pediatric associations have described their experience of making early surgical interventions, "There are situations for which any decision may lead to dissatisfaction."[59] Rather than categorizing such intractability as irrelevant to critique, then, I am going to place the difficult nature of treatment decisions center stage in my analysis.

To theorize difficulty, I would like to revisit and expand the theory of subjectivity that I introduced in chapter 2. To inhabit a position of subjectivity means assuming a vantage point from which one regards the world—a way of seeing that renders some things salient and others invisible or irrelevant. For instance, subjects in contemporary industrialized societies typically see female and male bodies as being starkly different, even though the majority of human body parts are not sexually dimorphic.[60] Inhabiting a subject position also means regarding oneself as possessing certain incontrovertible qualities and sensibilities— having a sense that one is "unique, (relatively) independent, and capable of making choices," as the political theorist Elizabeth Wingrove articulates it.[61] In this way, subjectivity is reflexive— the ability to reflect on oneself from a perspective that is one's own, as I phrased it in chapter 2. Despite this sense of singularity, the same subject position can be inhabited by many individuals; that is the positional nature of subjectivity. For example, in chapter 2 I discussed how children with intersex anatomies are positioned as gendered subjects of surgery, each seeing themselves as belonging to a gender. In the present chapter, I am interested in the subject position occupied by the adults who gather around those children. To describe the experience of these adults as subjective is not to imply that they are willfully biased; rather, it is to say that their actions lead them to inhabit a common vantage point. As clinicians, intersex support-group representatives, and commentators from other disciplines have all said, there is "a genuine struggle regarding appropriate care for children and families living with these conditions."[62] Taking their phrasing as my inspiration, I argue that adults who make decisions about childhood intersex surgery are positioned as subjects of struggle. This means that they occupy a subject position in which the use of surgery for intersex causes them to struggle.

To understand exactly why these subjects struggle, we need to step back from intersex medicine briefly and consider what it means to act in liquid modernity. This is a matter of how the social arrangements of the age inform the way we assign meanings to our actions, infusing practices of all kinds with a sense of ease or difficulty that is both historically situated and personally felt. Earlier I noted that liquid modernity is characterized by transient social relationships and everyday disorientation— the aftermath of a decline in collective experience that originated with the dispersal of heavy capitalism into postindustrial forms of production. The decline in collective experience has led to what Bauman calls "an individualized, privatized version of modernity."[63] Under such atomized social arrangements, the prevalent way to interpret our actions is according to personal intent, in particular the private conviction that one is acting in good faith. "We like our good intentions to constitute the meaning of our acts," Lauren Berlant has observed. Accordingly, Berlant adds, "we do not like to be held responsible for consequences we did not mean to enact."[64] So the degree of ease that we experience when we act reflects the extent to which the consequences coincide with our intentions. When the meaning of our actions diverges from what we intended, it feels correspondingly difficult—*Hey, that's not what I meant!* The strangeness of the body produced by intersex genital surgery is an exemplary instance of this divergence between intentions and consequences because the peculiar and unpredictable outcomes of surgery are at odds with the intent to normalize. Indeed, the very fact that medical power is open to reframing by critics and activists—as discipline, regulation, and erasure—demonstrates that medical intentions cannot dictate what the results of intersex surgery mean. I contend that the subject position of struggle arises from the impossibility of using such surgery to do what one intends.

Just as the contemporary medicalization of intersex is historically specific, so too is the subject position of struggle. It marks the problem of being an individual in liquid modernity who has to decide about genital surgery for intersex. In this respect, the subject position of struggle takes shape in a period in which surgical normalization is at once technically conceivable and routinely unachievable. To put it another way, the prospect of surgically normalizing the intersex body and the implausibility of doing so are aspects of the same historical formation. As a consequence, the practice of intersex surgery positions doctors and parents as subjects who are "capable of making choices," in Wingrove's phrase, yet whose choices cannot result in the genital normalization that they intend. Their struggle exists in the gap between their choice to use such interventions to normalize the intersex body and the strange outcomes of surgery. So even though liquid modernity creates the conditions for pervasive individualism, it also brings forth practices that cannot be explained by individual intentions. Clearly, then, it would be mistaken to restrict criticisms of intersex surgery to the normalization that such interventions intend to achieve. For example, Cary Gabriel Costello has criticized intersex surgeries on the basis that they are "intended to enforce the ideology that bodies of nonbinary sex are unacceptable."[65] This overstates the extent to which intentions control surgical outcomes. Regardless of how strongly doctors and parents may like to enforce the ideology that Costello criticizes, they would also say that they are not enforcing much at all: they are instead wrestling with their own incapability to make sex binary. I think therefore that an acute discrepancy exists between the exercise of medical power through genital surgery on children and the "genuine struggle" that adults go through when making decisions about it. At stake in this discrepancy is an underlying question of whether the subject position of struggle is also a position of power.

For subjects of struggle, the answer to this question is no. For them, there is a self-evident line of sight that connects failures of surgical normalization to their own powerlessness to make treatment decisions that go as intended. It is obvious to these subjects that they lack power: the strangeness and unpredictability of the postsurgical body proves it. Indeed, doctors and parents do not need anyone to tell them that they should worry about surgical interventions; they worry by themselves. In a seminal essay on subjectivity, the philosopher Louis Althusser once argued that every subject is "endowed with a consciousness in which he freely forms or freely recognizes ideas in which he believes."[66] I mentioned earlier that inhabiting a position of subjectivity means assuming a vantage point on the world as well as on oneself. When subjects struggle over intersex treatment decisions, they freely form the idea that the world contains intractable problems of normalization ("situations for which any decision may lead to dissatisfaction") just as they freely recognize themselves as being disempowered to respond ("living with massive dilemmas"). In this regard, subjects act autonomously despite the historically contingent nature of their position. However, the obviousness of what subjects see is a matter of perspective. In light of my analysis in this chapter, I argue that adults around the patient do have power—the power to make the intersex body strange. By stepping aside from the subject position of struggle and conceptualizing the action of medical power separately from the content of individual intentions, we can discern that power is exercised by *not* achieving the genital normalization that subjects intend. In other words, their power to make the body strange comes from the very fact that their treatment decisions do not unfold as intended. Subjects of struggle cannot see this because from their perspective the power to make the body strange is experienced—freely, autonomously, as Althusser says—as the struggle of making it normal.

I am arguing that at the subject position of struggle, medical power assumes the mantle of powerlessness. The subjective experience of disempowerment obscures the fact that doctors and parents wield real power to make intersex bodies strange through surgical wounding. In the apparent absence of power, the strange results of genital surgery are transformed into reasons for subjects to worry rather than into occasions to criticize medical power over intersex bodies. I suggest, therefore, that the subject position of struggle is medical power's alibi. Earlier I described subjectivity as a way of seeing that renders some things salient and others invisible; in this case, the salience of the struggle renders medical power invisible to those who possess it. Despite this illusion of powerlessness, though, there is nothing imaginary about the struggle that subjects experience. Their struggle to normalize the intersex body is "a historical event," in the words of Wingrove's commentary on subject formation: It arises through the exercise of real medical power in a specific historical period.[67] At the same time, their struggle immerses subjects in what Althusser calls "a non-historical reality," which is their subjective powerlessness.[68] So although it may seem like treatment decisions are "difficult and stressful" because they are made by subjects who are powerless, actually the reverse is true. These subjects see themselves as powerless because their treatment decisions are a struggle. In this way, the self-reflection at the heart of subjectivity explains how a struggle can be "genuine" even while it engenders a distorted vantage point on what is really happening—the use of medical power to make intersex bodies stranger and stranger.[69] At this point in my chapter, readers might ask why doctors and parents do not simply abandon the idea of using surgery to normalize intersex bodies, given how difficult they find it. Sometimes they do. In the coda that follows, though, I am going to show how medical power can endure even in decisions that are taken to avoid intersex surgery.

PRIVACY AND PREJUDICE

My inquiry into the nature of medical power in this chapter has shown that medicalization and medical power do not operate in lockstep when it comes to intersex. Far from it. The power of intersex medicine in late-modern times has a decidedly off-kilter relationship with the medicalization of intersex. Over the course of this chapter, I have revealed that the boundaries of medical power cannot easily be framed because its operation is streaked with failure; that medical power is entangled with bodies that simultaneously enable and thwart its passage; and that the exercise of medical power grants doctors and parents privileged knowledge, even as it instills chronic uncertainty regarding the treatment decisions they make. In all these ways, medical power over intersex assumes a fragile and elusive form that is antithetical to the intensity and visibility of medicalization yet that prolongs the medicalization of intersex and disempowerment of patients, nonetheless. I have revealed, too, that the exercise of power is concealed by the difficulties encountered by doctors and parents: we have seen how their struggle hides from them the power that they possess to make the body strange through genital surgery. However, medical power does not vanish completely. That is because the strange wounds of the postsurgical body betray the operation of power. In this coda to the chapter, I want to examine how medical power reaches its vanishing point in a different treatment for intersex in which genital surgery is not done at all. The treatment to which I am referring is preimplantation genetic testing (PGT) to avert the birth of children with intersex characteristics through in vitro fertilization (IVF).[70] PGT for intersex entails the use of genetic screening to identify embryos that have the potential to develop into intersex bodies. Those embryos are then discarded. Only embryos that are believed not to harbor intersex characteristics are retained for implantation. I am going to argue that the practice of PGT perfects the disappearance of medical power by removing such power from public scrutiny.

The use of IVF is a prerequisite for PGT because testing takes place while embryos are in the laboratory, but uptake of PGT is not limited to parents who require IVF to conceive. Some choose IVF specifically for the opportunity to undertake PGT.[71] In relation to intersex, PGT accomplishes what genital surgery cannot: normalization without complications. "Although surgery may fail to produce a body of the nominated sex," the philosopher Robert Sparrow has observed, PGT results in children who "will almost always be born with the desired chromosomal, endocrinological, and anatomical sex."[72] In this regard, PGT is not merely a means to avoid intersex; crucially, it is also a means to avoid genital surgery.[73] As Sparrow explains, "Questions about the possibility of surgical and/or psychological harms to the individual being 'treated,' which loom so large in the context of the debate about surgery for intersex conditions, do not arise in the context of genetic selection."[74] By enabling embryos to be discarded before they develop intersex characteristics, PGT bypasses difficult decisions about surgery. Therefore, when potential parents use PGT to avoid doing intersex surgery, they alleviate a struggle that has not yet occurred. The theoretical framework that I have developed in this chapter provides an original way to analyze this phenomenon. I argue that these potential parents identify with the subject position of struggle. They act as though they already face a decision to do normalizing surgery that is going to fail. Even with no child and no surgery yet, the positional nature of subjectivity means that potential parents can assume the same vantage point as existing parents whose real children undergo surgical interventions. To put this another way, the practice of PGT leads individuals to identify with a position that is not their own. Unlike genital surgery, however, PGT offers relief from the struggle. The preemptive disposal of embryos circumvents the strangeness and unpredictability of the postsurgical body. PGT thereby grants potential parents the prospect of achieving exactly the normalization that they intend.

Some critical commentators have objected to PGT on the grounds that its "normalizing power" exacerbates prejudice against existing individuals with intersex anatomies, contributing to social hostility toward genital atypicality.[75] In a strident counterargument to these objections, the philosopher Laurence McCullough has asserted that PGT is not at all discriminatory, provided that potential parents and medical staff keep its use to themselves, ensuring that it "will never become public."[76] McCullough claims, in other words, that PGT to prevent intersex births is a private matter. When construed as a wholly private process, very little seems to happen in the disposal of embryos through PGT other than a discreet release of pressure from the potential parents' consciences. The moment of normalization is marked only by their sense of relief at having averted a difficult future. So whereas the disappearance of medical power in the struggle over genital surgery can never be absolute because the postsurgical body bears the signs of power's operation, in PGT the exercise of power recedes into privacy. Yet, contrary to what McCullough claims, for this very reason I think that keeping PGT private exacerbates prejudice. This is because it creates a social world in which the elimination of intersex births constitutes a choice that is not considered worthy of public discourse. The lack of discussion means, in turn, that potential parents cannot be held to account for their decisions.[77] In the purest expression of Bauman's insight that "the prime technique of power is now escape, slippage, elision and avoidance," the use of medical power in the practice of PGT evades public scrutiny. I argue that the bloodless action of power in the disposal of embryos to avoid later genital surgery is the vanishing point where the idea of surgery for intersex penetrates subjects so deeply that it achieves its own negation. Although most criticisms of intersex medicine are preoccupied with arguing against surgeries taking place in the present day, it is in the privacy of decisions to do PGT that surgeries that have never happened are quietly reshaping the membership of the late-modern social world.

6

WAS INTERSEX REAL?

O ne of my earliest publications on intersex was an article titled "Is Intersexuality Real?" in 2001. My answer
to the question was *no, but it's complicated*. I posed the
question to emphasize that atypical genitalia are constructed in
mainstream Western culture and medicine as not merely ambiguously sexed but also less than fully real. Drawing on feminist
science studies and critical theory, my argument was that all
knowledge is constructed, but not all constructions appear to be
equally real. Whereas femaleness and maleness are constructed
as real states of being—permanent, natural, and irreducible—
intersex (or *intersexuality* as it also used to be called) is constructed
as a temporary or counterfeit state, ready to be constructed away
to reveal female or male anatomies that are unfinished or hidden.[1]
This chapter will pick up the task of analyzing how the realness of
intersex takes shape through diagnostic knowledge about the
body by considering how the introduction of new language for
atypical sex development has affected both medical practice and
activism since 2001. The chapter will also serve as a metacom-
mentary on the role of critique: I aim to demonstrate that it
remains vitally important to deconstruct intersex medicine at a
time when health professionals, patients, families, and activists

are—according to some stakeholders—all working together and talking a common language.

FROM KNIVES TO WORDS

Diagnostic language matters. In the light of work by Alice Dreger in the late 1990s on the history of medical nomenclature, I suggested in "Is Intersexuality Real?" that the diagnoses *true hermaphrodite* and *pseudohermaphrodite* characterized intersex bodies as either rare or inauthentic.[2] Originating in the nineteenth century, these diagnostic terms remained in circulation when I wrote this article at the turn of the twenty-first century. Typified by a mixture of ovarian and testicular tissue, so-called true hermaphroditism has always been highly unusual, so the effect of naming it the true form of sexual ambiguity was to rarify and exoticize intersex.[3] This turned true hermaphroditism into a colonial curiosity, spurring racist medical efforts to find cases among nonwhite communities outside the West.[4] Moreover, because the gonads in true hermaphroditism usually do not function, to call this state *true* was to cast intersex bodies as nonfunctional by default. Pseudohermaphroditism, where either ovaries or testes are present and may be functional, is more common. Yet the prefix *pseudo-* insinuated that such bodies are not really intersex but can instead be classified as female or male on the basis of their gonads. Accordingly, this diagnosis was typically formulated as either *female pseudohermaphroditism* for those with ovaries or *male pseudohermaphroditism* for those with testes. Ostensibly, the terminology of true and pseudohermaphroditism distinguished between types of intersex, but I think it also did something else: It portrayed all types of intersex as dubiously real by invoking a prior difference between female and male gonads. In this way, the language of true and pseudohermaphroditism sustained a hierarchy between types of sexual difference that are real (differentiated by gonads) and those that are not (differentiated by intersex characteristics). In "Is Intersexuality Real?" I proposed the alternative terms *hermaphroditic pseudofemale* and *hermaphroditic pseudomale* to flip this hierarchy by prioritizing intersex characteristics. I wanted to let the presence of intersex body parts put in doubt the realness of female and male features rather than the other way around.

In my advocacy of alternative language, I joined contemporary commentators on medicine who were arguing for the expansion of discourse about intersex. Authors such as Cheryl Chase, Milton Diamond, Anne Fausto-Sterling, Morgan Holmes, and Suzanne Kessler—as well as Dreger—were calling variously for more patient testimonies, wider media coverage, broader multidisciplinary scholarship, increased psychological counseling, and greater dialogue between support groups and patients, families, and clinicians—all types of discourse that differed from traditional diagnostic language about intersex.[5] At the time, it seemed that "medical interventions on children with an ambiguous sex are already an old story; what is new is that we now talk about them," one sociologist remarked in the same year as "Is Intersexuality Real?"[6] But the diversification of intersex discourse was never intended as a mere commentary on traditional treatment. For those of us in favor of treatment reform, the practice of giving clinical, scholarly, and popular attention to a range of discourses on intersex was the right thing to do—a better response to genital diversity than the performance of childhood surgery and its purported foreclosure of discussion about sexual ambiguity. In Kessler's explanation, "There are many ways to make parents comfortable with children. One way, the one currently preferred by intersex surgeons, is to use surgery to make the child look normal to the parents. Another is to use language to achieve this same purpose." Talking about variant genitals in a nonstigmatizing way held the promise of transforming the perception of intersex from an untenable, unreal state into a real and lovable kind of sexual difference. Kessler eloquently described such a change as a choice between knives and words.[7] In this sense, critics did not want just to talk about medical treatment but also to replace it with talking.

Against this backdrop, a group of critics including Chase and Dreger went on to publish a paper in 2005 that admonished the terminology of *true hermaphroditism* and *pseudohermaphroditism* as "illogical, outdated, and harmful." In its place, they recommended "specific etiology-based diagnoses" that would no longer prioritize gonads in the definition of sexual difference. Their focus on etiology implied that better diagnostic language rather than the wholesale rejection of medical discourse might usefully draw attention to the particularities of individual sexual development—for example, by specifying that a person is insensitive to androgens produced by their testes as opposed to diagnosing the person as a male pseudohermaphrodite on the basis of those gonads. In closing their paper, the authors briefly put forward *disorders of sexual differentiation* as an umbrella term for the various diagnoses that might supersede *true hermaphrodite* and *pseudohermaphrodite*.[8] In the following year, the same authors were among the contributors to a pair of handbooks for clinicians and families. Both handbooks advocated the reform of medical treatment, including a halt to genital cosmetic surgery in infancy.[9] In the handbooks, diagnoses such as *true hermaphrodite* and *pseudohermaphrodite* were subsumed into a slightly different umbrella phrase, *disorders of sex development*. Explaining to handbook contributors this change of wording from *sexual differentiation* to *sex development*, coordinating editor Dreger wrote that the former phrase misled clinicians into thinking that it referred only to gonads—that is, to the differentiation of gonads into ovaries or testes—and therefore did not fix the problem that it was intended to solve. Contrastingly, *disorders of sex development* encompassed more than gonadal differentiation.[10] Another important change in language separated the handbooks from the earlier article. The journal article never recommended *disorders of sexual differentiation* as a replacement for the words *intersex* and *intersexuality*. But throughout the handbooks, *disorders of sex development* replaced both those words.

Clinical uptake of the phrase *disorders of sex development*, abbreviated to DSD, was swift. It was quickened by the fact that preparation of the handbooks coincided with a conference organized by the major European and American pediatric endocrinology professional societies. Late in 2005, some fifty leading clinicians met to review treatment protocols for intersex.[11] One of two patient advocates also invited to the conference, Chase distributed drafts of the handbooks to participants.[12] Chase's aspiration was that the DSD terminology would be "really appealing to doctors," encouraging their engagement with the treatment-reform recommendations contained in the handbooks.[13] In transforming the language used by clinicians, Chase was effective. Medics at the conference embraced *DSD* as an umbrella term, defining it as "congenital conditions in which development of chromosomal, gonadal or anatomical sex is atypical."[14] On the grounds that "gender labeling in the diagnosis should be avoided" but that genetics should be specified where possible, conference participants delineated new categories beneath the umbrella term—such as "46,XY DSD" in place of "male pseudohermaphroditism," "46,XX DSD" in place of "female pseudohermaphroditism," and "ovotesticular DSD" for what was previously called "true hermaphroditism."[15] Like the handbooks, they advanced this terminology to supersede not only the word *hermaphrodite* but also the word *intersex* in diagnoses. Echoing a claim in the handbooks that such older words appeared "frightening and imprecise" to affected individuals and families, medics at the conference rejected both *hermaphrodite* and *intersex* as "confusing" and "potentially pejorative."[16] They asserted that DSD diagnoses, in contrast, were "understandable" and "psychologically sensitive" to those affected.[17] The output of the conference was a collaboratively written policy statement addressing both nomenclature and treatment and published in leading American and European pediatrics journals in 2006.[18] The statement's impact on medical terminology was striking. Two years after its publication, the use of *intersex* as a diagnosis in medical literature had fallen by 50 percent, supplanted by *disorders of sex development*.[19]

Criticisms of the change in terminology emerged rapidly, too, starting with objections by some contributors in the handbooks themselves.[20] Centering on the use of the word *disorder*, complaints fell into two broad groups. Some commentators accepted the premise that diagnostic language should be revised to facilitate treatment reform but objected to the characterization of certain types of sex development as disordered. These commentators proposed alternative diagnostic language in which atypical sex development would be described as being *divergent, different, discordant*, or *diverse*—all options that would allow continued use of the acronym DSD—or as being *variations of sex development* or *variations of reproductive development*, under the acronyms VSD and VRD.[21] Though more neutral in tone than *disorder*, the assorted alternatives still upheld the principle that medical knowledge about sex development is possible and useful. Other critics of the DSD terminology argued against diagnostic language entirely. To these commentators, the problem was not primarily the word *disorder*, as though the selection of a differ-ent word might make the problem go away, but rather the authority of clinicians to name bodies in the first place. In this view, *disorder* was emblematic of medical power. More than a poor choice of word, it was a symbol of how clinicians could decide which words apply to other people's bodies. These critics preferred the retention of *intersex*.[22] An additional group of com-mentators adopted a mixed position, either by employing a combination of *DSD* and *intersex* or by leaving the first letter of the acronym DSD open to interpretation to mean *disorders* or *differences*.[23] The range of reactions to the terminological shift unsettled Kessler's earlier distinction between knives and words in the management of intersex. Whereas for Kessler the use of words could be a progressive alternative to the use of knives, the fractured responses to DSD revealed that some new ways of talking about intersex might not be progressive after all.

Was intersex real, then? Although the turn away from the language of hermaphroditism promised to make variant geni-tals more real by decentering the gonadal definition of sexual difference, the result of this move was the withdrawal of the terms *intersex* and *intersexuality* from most medical discourse. I had argued in 2001 that intersex was constructed as less than fully real, a state that could be constructed away to reveal female-ness or maleness. After 2006, it seemed as if intersex had been constructed away to reveal disorders of sex development, described by Chase as "the underlying physiology that causes the atypical sex anatomy."[24] Looking back, I think there are two broad ways to theorize what happened—as change or as conti-nuity. Theorized the first way, the adoption of DSD has cata-lyzed a departure from traditional medical treatment, albeit not from medicalization. Theorized the second way, the adop-tion of DSD has furthered the traditional medical project of making intersex disappear. By the second interpretation, the new terminology has done what surgery always sought to do—make intersex unreal. In the sections that follow in this chapter, I will focus on evaluating whether the emergence of DSD was a moment of change or continuity in the history of intersex and its medicalization. I am going to make an original argument that pushes beyond the usual parameters of the debate about DSD to consider a topic that is widely ignored but crucial to the very idea of managing genital variations: the social structure of work.

DIAGNOSING IDENTITIES

The question of whether the adoption of the term *DSD* changes anything pivots for many commentators on whether diagnostic language determines the identities of patients. In the article that made the case for discarding the terminology of hermaphroditism in 2005, Dreger, Chase, and their coauthors criticized the existing diagnostic language not only for its representation of sexually ambiguous body parts but also for its representation of people. Their complaint centered on the depiction of patients as hermaphrodites. By their account, the prevailing practice of naming "the whole person according to the condition" conferred on affected individuals all the negative overtones of the diagnosis—spurious, nonfunctional, and outlandishly rare.[25] The terminology of hermaphroditism thereby constructed "a problematic type of person," as Ellen Feder and Katrina Karkazis phrased it in a later commentary.[26] Likewise, to describe persons as being intersex or intersexual could insinuate doubt over their gender and sexual identities, Dreger and April Herndon noted subsequently.[27] When clinicians at the 2005 conference criticized the use of *hermaphrodite* and *intersex*, they took up these arguments against the use of "all-encompassing" terms to label patients.[28] For those who see the introduction of the term *DSD* as a catalyst for the transformation of medical practice, the new terminology usefully separates diagnosis from identity. This is because, unlike both *hermaphrodite* and *intersex*, it names the bodily characteristics that patients have instead of the types of people that patients are. A disorder of sex development, Feder and Karkazis have written, "is a medical condition, not an identity."[29] The change of terminology therefore discourages doctors from unwarranted speculation about the identities of affected individuals. It gives them a better way to think about their patients not as sexually ambiguous people but as regular "human beings with a diagnosis."[30] Arguably then, changing the relationship between diagnosis and identity can improve the practice of medicine by reducing bias and mission creep.

Critics of the designation *DSD*, too, are alert to the relationship between diagnostic language and the identities of patients. However, they diverge from authors such as Chase and Dreger by arguing against the transformative power of DSD. The basis for this argument varies between critics. To some critics, the new terminology fails to separate diagnosis from identity because it constructs its own problematic type of person—a disordered person instead of a hermaphrodite. From this perspective, the diagnosis of a disorder of sex development casts affected individuals as being "wrong" or "inherently dysfunctional."[31] David Cameron, a handbook contributor who objected to the new language, has explained that "I don't like negative medical terms defining me."[32] Critics such as Cameron reject the new terminology on the grounds that it defines people, not conditions; for them, the term *DSD* is the wrong answer to Chase and Dreger's call for diagnostic language that would "label the condition rather than the person."[33] Other critics decline this call altogether. They object not to the construction of any particular type of person but to the construction of atypical sex as a condition. For example, the activist Lynnell Stephani Long has recounted that before the introduction of DSD, "when people asked me about my 'condition' I told them I had no 'condition': I am Intersex."[34] From this perspective, the separation between identity and diagnosis that might be achieved by the replacement of *intersex* with *disorders of sex development* is unwelcome. In contrast to the view that diagnostic language ought not to define individuals at all, for critics like Long the terminological change overlooks the fact that in diagnostic language "individuals *are* being portrayed rather than just medical disorders."[35] To use such language purely to label conditions is therefore a failure to recognize the identities of those affected. In summary, critics vary over whether they object to the term *DSD* for the ascription of the identity "disordered" or for the removal of the identity "intersex."[36] Whether they think the introduction of *DSD* has failed or succeeded in parting diagnosis from identity, they are skeptical that the new language is a change from medical tradition.

The diversity of positions regarding the relationship between diagnostic language and patient identities shows that this relationship cannot easily be described. To describe the relationship is to take a position on it, and no position is agreeable to all commentators. They agree, at least, that diagnostic language ought not to confer a bad identity on any patient. But there is no concord over what constitutes a bad identity. I think this lack of concord is inevitable because all identities can change in meaning. To take up even a pejorative term as one's identity is not to endorse the term's existing connotations; rather, it is to challenge those connotations through the very act of identification and thereby to alter the meaning of the identity.[37] The clinical term *intersex*, which activists in the 1990s recast as an identity, exemplifies this point. Hence, I disagree with some opponents of the term *DSD* who fear that diagnoses can become "static symbols" of "inferiority" that affected individuals "might shoulder for a lifetime."[38] Identities are not static; no identity is irreversibly bad simply because it originates in a diagnosis. In the same way, no identity is indelibly good, either, so there can be no concord between commentators about the line between good and bad identities. Some might argue that this difference of views would be irrelevant if everyone could agree on the separation of identity from diagnostic language. However, I think agreement on that, too, is impossible. To distinguish the DSD terminology from the language of identity, Feder has suggested that the terminology names conditions that are "merely incidental to one's person."[39] This suggestion, however, underplays the significance that conditions can have. As participants at the 2005 conference put it, DSDs can be "chronic medical conditions with life-long consequences." How one lives with a chronic condition can indeed be a matter of identity—good or bad.[40] Therefore, unanimity between commentators cannot be built around the idea that medical conditions are incidental to identity.

Despite holding irreconcilable viewpoints, I think commentators are alike in one respect: they all make assumptions about the body. They argue from the premise of a natural body that exists prior to medical treatment, which grounds their claims about the remit of diagnostic language. Given that their arguments diverge about the remit of diagnostic language, the meaning of the natural body differs between commentators, too. For some, it means the body that has a condition. Naturalized as the object of medical diagnosis, this body is the location of what Chase calls "the underlying physiology that causes the atypical sex anatomy." For others, the natural body means the atypical sex anatomy itself, not its underlying cause. This body is the ground for identity claims; it is the foundation for Long's assertion "I am Intersex." These two examples show how opposing claims can arise from different assumptions about a common premise, the natural body. But when the stakes of the debate are set by the body that exists prior to treatment, commentators on all sides struggle to account for the body that has undergone treatment. Medically modified, this body is no longer describable as natural. Rather, it is constructed—the product of interventions that aim to make sexual ambiguity go away. As I have explored throughout this book, such interventions do not make the body straightforwardly sexually unambiguous. They have lasting effects that are disfiguring and disorienting. So even though the 2005 conference participants hoped to identify and alleviate "chronic medical conditions with life-long consequences," clinical interventions often create long-term conditions of their own, including hormonal deficiencies after gonadectomy, urethral strictures after penile surgery, and disturbed tactility after clitoral reduction.[41] I believe that neither the "underlying physiology" posited by Chase nor the physical characteristics that enable Long to say "I am Intersex" can be untangled from such effects. Because treatment leaves the body in weirdly constructed states, this outcome problematizes all arguments premised upon the natural body.

The question of whether the DSD terminology is a point of change or continuity in the history of intersex cannot be settled by establishing whether patient identities are determined by the diagnoses applied to our bodies. I have shown in this section that there are multiple reasons why this is so—identities cannot be sorted into good and bad; conditions cannot be separated from identities; and neither conditions nor identities can be unraveled from the effects of medical treatment upon the body. Many writers on DSD have dwelled on the relationship between diagnostic language and patient identities, but their shared interest has not given rise to a mutual understanding of what that relationship means, what it should be, or whether it should exist at all. I think this ambivalence is unavoidable. Its effect is that we cannot establish the significance that new diagnostic language such as *DSD* has for identity, so we cannot know whether the term *DSD* changes anything. For that insight, we must look elsewhere. In this section, I have argued that although commentators disagree with each other, they all have difficulty in accounting for the body constructed by treatment. This suggests that by addressing the medical construction of the body, we might find a way to step around the existing positions in the DSD debate. We already know that medical treatment constructs patient bodies, but that is not the full picture. In the next section, I want to consider the bodies that clinicians inhabit and what they do with them. Moving beyond the imponderable conferral of identities upon patients whose bodies are diagnosed and treated, this is a matter of how the embodied acts of diagnosing and treating DSDs define medical professionals.

MAKING MEDICAL PEOPLE

The policy statement that followed the 2005 conference advocated changing the way atypical sex characteristics are diagnosed and treated, not just by introducing new terms but also by altering how and when clinicians make decisions. Whereas affected infants were traditionally assigned to a gender as promptly as possible according to the surgical ease with which their genitals could be made to seem female or male, the statement advised a slower decision-making process unpropelled by surgical considerations.

It recommended that gender assignments "must be avoided prior to expert evaluation in newborns" and stipulated that both this diagnostic evaluation and subsequent treatments should be done by "an experienced multidisciplinary team."[42] Challenging the idea that surgeons have sufficient expertise to assign gender, the statement made consultation across disciplines the standard for good practice. It proposed the involvement of specialists from "endocrinology, surgery and/or urology, psychology/psychiatry, gynaecology, genetics, neonatology and, if available, social work, nursing and medical ethics." It also encouraged the participation of patients and families in making decisions with the multidisciplinary team.[43] The statement received criticism, however, for overstating the potential for such teamwork to achieve change. According to the sociologist and patient advocate Georgiann Davis, the multidisciplinary team envisaged by the policy statement is both too large and insufficiently diverse. Though team members may privately debate treatment options and admit uncertainty, the size of the team can give to patients and families an impression of comprehensive authority and certainty, thus deterring them from seeking alternative opinions or giving their own opinion. Further, because such a team is composed mostly of people from clinical disciplines, its members remain unlikely to give serious consideration to social explanations for gender, sex, and sexuality or to discuss these explanations with patients and families. The combined result of these factors is that the advice provided by multidisciplinary teams may be oversimplified and unduly medicalized, Davis argues.[44] Other critics have argued similarly that the proliferation of disciplines involved in diagnosis and treatment does not diffuse medical authority but sustains or even intensifies it.[45]

Davis's critique highlights that simply adding or changing specialisms in a multidisciplinary team may not improve care for affected individuals. Indeed, the policy statement recognized the need for team members to undertake dedicated training and to educate other professionals with whom the team interacts.[46] A follow-up policy statement in 2016 advocated greater shared responsibility between disciplines for the clinical decisions made by teams.[47] Regardless of whether one is sympathetic or skeptical toward the approach recommended by the original statement, I think that multidisciplinary teams embody ideas about work that deserve critical scrutiny. At base, the diagnosis and treatment of affected individuals require effort. The amount of effort required is in part a reflection of the terminological change from *intersex* to *DSD*. Because the new terminology provides more etiologically descriptive diagnoses than were common previously, it increases the obligation on medical professionals to "employ precision when applying definitions and diagnostic labels," as the original statement puts it.[48] Such precision takes time to achieve; hence, a delay in gender assignment can occur while work is underway. Types of diagnostic work on newborns described by the statement include genetic testing, physical examination, ultrasound imaging, and six types of biochemical test.[49] All are specialized kinds of work—instances of what social theorists have called the division of labor.[50] Dividing labor into different specialisms—here genetics, pediatrics, radiology, and biochemistry—is a prerequisite for the formation of multidisciplinary teams. But when we assume that disciplines are the building blocks of an effective response to sexual ambiguity, we risk placing the division of labor itself beyond critique. In other words, even if the composition of multidisciplinary teams can challenge the historical dominance of surgery in clinical decisions, the specialization of work into disciplines is likely to go unquestioned.

The lack of critical attention to the division of labor is especially clear in discussions about the role that psychology should play in multidisciplinary teams. The policy statement mandated that "psychosocial care provided by mental health staff" must be "an integral part of management"—and even be "at the heart" of how teams treat affected individuals, as one of the lead authors elaborated.[51] This requirement implies that the discipline of psychology is uniquely capable of transforming practice as opposed to being merely one specialism among others in an expanded team. Accordingly, some see the inclusion of psychologists in multidisciplinary teams as evidence that medical practice has changed following the introduction of the DSD terminology. One leading British team has argued that the presence of a psychologist shows that the whole team recognizes that physical and psychological care are interrelated.[52] Nevertheless, the follow-up statement of 2016 conceded that psychology in DSD treatment and research is typically characterized as being either solely about gender in the brain or a vague placeholder for all social and psychological concerns.[53] The use of psychology as a passive "emotional repository" has received criticism from the psychologist Lih-Mei Liao and the patient advocate Margaret Simmonds, who have observed that psychologists often lack the power to challenge clinical decisions despite their participation in multidisciplinary teams. Liao and Simmonds are among a group of critics who propose more wide-ranging and subversive roles for psychologists, from facilitating overall team development and training participants from other disciplines to interrogating how clinicians think and scrutinizing the ways in which psychological concepts are used to justify medical interventions.[54] However, none of these proposed roles, for all their innovative aspects, I argue, puts in question the division of labor. They just alter the labor assigned to psychologists. Like the original policy statement, these proposals cast psychology as a uniquely transformative discipline, and so in this respect they maintain the assumption that the problem of achieving medical change is solvable by specialization.

In my view, to specialize in any given discipline is to adopt ways of moving and touching that are discipline specific. Specialization is embodied. Patients are not the only bodies in the clinical encounter, but this fact is generally overlooked: In acts of diagnosis and treatment, the bodies of multidisciplinary team members labor over those of their patients. Moving differently according to their specializations, the different members touch patient bodies in distinct ways, varying from manual palpation and dilation to mediated interactions such as the slithery touch of the ultrasound transducer and the graze of the needle. Through differences in movement and touch, labor is divided between the bodies of team members. Specialization also means learning how to touch the tools that construct forms of knowledge specific to one's discipline—the geneticist does not palpate the patient, for example, but touches the apparatus of analysis to create diagnostic information from cellular samples. The opposition between knives and words that Kessler invoked is a contrast between tools as well. The tools of surgery differ from those of psychology, so these disciplines make distinctive demands on the bodies of practitioners. Some bodies labor with knives; others labor with words. In a multidisciplinary team, then, each body's discipline-specific movements distinguish its labor from the labor of others. As disciplines change, these differences vary, but the division of labor remains. What is more, calls to transform medical practice are assimilated into the division of labor so that discipline-specific types of work continue to be prevalent. This is exemplified by the transformative role assigned to psychology: Criticisms of surgery not only have driven the addition of psychology to multidisciplinary teams but also have become psychology's own specialty—the labor of critique. Fewer knives mean more words rather than less work. The division of labor always gives bodies something to do.

Cultural critics are accustomed to thinking of gender as a "corporeal style" following Judith Butler's analysis in *Gender Trouble* (1990), but I say that we should consider the embodied qualities of multidisciplinary labor as corporeal styles, too. For a member of a multidisciplinary team to represent a discipline is to move in a corporeal style separate from the styles of one's coworkers. Butler argued in *Gender Trouble* that corporeal styles imply the existence of an abiding self, which motivates behavior and is expressed by it. For Butler, the self does not precede the style, but the style makes it seem that way.[55] With this in mind, we can revisit the policy statement's apparently self-evident recommendation that patient bodies ought to undergo "expert evaluation." Being an expert such as a surgeon or a psychologist indicates fluency in a corporeal style—the authority, comfort, and legibility with which one's embodied movements evaluate and treat patients according to the conventions of a given discipline. After Butler, however, I would turn this observation around. It is fluency in a corporeal style that suggests the presence of an expert self who drives the stylized movements of the body. That is to say, the performance of specialized work implies the existence of a type of person, the expert, behind the work. This normalizes work as an expression of the self, so that specialization seems to originate in the expert rather than in the division of labor. The latter is both sustained and camouflaged by the idea that types of people preexist the specialized work that they perform. Therefore, I think it would be a mistake to assess

change in medical treatment by whether particular experts are
included in multidisciplinary teams. "Expert evaluation" sounds
uncontentious, but dividing labor between experts frames the
question of continuity or change in the management of atypical
sex as an issue of who should be working rather than *whether
work should be done at all*. The latter is the deeper question I want
to address in the next section.

WORKING TOGETHER

Changing medical practice could mean working differently.
Alternatively, it could mean ceasing to work. Its meaning
depends on whether we believe work to be the right response to
atypical sex characteristics. This is a foundational question to
which commentators have opposing answers. For some critics of
traditional treatment, the answer is straightforward: work is the
wrong response, so doing work differently not only misrecog-
nizes the nature of the problem but perpetuates it. For example,
altering the type of clitoral reduction performed on infants does
not make infant clitoral surgery an acceptable practice, even if
some medics may regard the results as technically superior to
previous interventions. As Dreger has remarked, "All the evidence in the world in favor of the 'effectiveness' of a treatment
doesn't make it ethical."[56] From this standpoint, the distribution
of work between disciplines is an overcomplicated distraction
from "key ethical and human rights concerns," in the words of
the patient advocate Morgan Carpenter.[57] Irrespective of the
composition of the team performing the work, at stake are issues
such as consent, fertility, and bodily integrity. This universal-
izing critique contrasts to the argument made by clinical commentators who see work as the right response to atypical sex.

Following the policy statement published in 2006, it has become common for doctors to advise that the work of diagnosis, treatment, and disclosure should be done in a case-by-case way. Whereas critics such as Dreger and Carpenter appeal to principles that apply across treatments, teams, and patients, many doctors reject what they call "generalized statements" in favor of "a more individualized approach to each case."[58] For instance, when an international group of clinicians was challenged in 2016 to recognize the right of all patients to decide whether to have healthy genital tissue removed, they countered that it is "wrong to amalgamate completely different situations" because "each DSD patient is an individual."[59] In this case-by-case approach, changing medical practice simply means working differently for each patient—not ceasing work for all patients.

But there is a problem with the case-by-case approach: By default, *all* cases receive medical treatment, so the approach is only superficially tailored to each case.[60] Characterizing atypical sexual features as disordered, the term *DSD* discourages a genuinely case-by-case approach in favor of a treatment-by-treatment response to each disorder diagnosed. Making such treatment individualized does not allow for cases in which affected individuals may not want clinical interventions or might not require them. For doctors who believe that work is the right response to atypical sex, the possibility of withholding medical treatment seems like no response at all—a failure to act rather than a different choice of action. Doctors therefore routinely categorize the deferral of treatment beyond childhood as "doing nothing," contrasting it to early clinical interventions that they define implicitly as doing something.[61] On one side of this contrast are activities that count as work, which seem to do something. On the other side are activities that are not work, which appear not to do anything. This opposition is contrived but influential nonetheless. Critics have warned that when options are presented to parents as a choice between doing something and doing nothing, parents are primed to select the former.[62] By selecting early medical treatments, parents feel as if they are taking positive action on behalf of their children. So even though medical advocates of the case-by-case approach recommend creating for each patient "an individual plan best arrived at by a multidisciplinary team in concert with the parents," the conversations that shape such plans are far from neutral.[63] In this context, childhood surgery can appeal to parents precisely because it is irreversible; the fact that it cannot be undone makes it seem like the most decisive means to get something done.

Perhaps, yes, we ought to do something but do it better. If the problem is that treatment plans remain skewed toward early surgical interventions, then the solution may be to make better plans. We might start by overhauling the portrayal of treatment options that do not involve childhood surgery so that they are no longer depicted as indecisive or passive. Instead of signaling indecision, the deferral of surgery beyond childhood could be understood as a purposeful course of action to secure patient consent in the future. Likewise, psychological care without early surgery could be recognized as an "alternative active pathway for children and parents to allow them to meet the challenges posed by having a genital appearance different to expectation," as the psychologist Julie Alderson and the gynecologist Naomi Crouch have argued.[64] Changing what it means to do something in response to variant genitalia would reorient conversations between parents and medical professionals away from surgical options, while still allowing them to feel that they are taking action—pursuing an "active pathway," in Alderson and Crouch's phrase. Treatment plans could also be made better by widening participation. In a pathbreaking move, the policy statement of

2006 acknowledged formally that "support groups complement the work of the health care team and, together, can help improve services." Describing support groups and medical professionals as "partners," the statement called for dialogue and collaboration between them.[65] The involvement of patient support groups in conversations about treatment could guide parents and clinical teams to make more rounded choices: for example, they may be more circumspect about long-term treatment outcomes after consulting with affected adults. If support groups became regular partners in the creation of treatment plans, and if "doing something about genital atypicality" were no longer synonymous with "doing surgery," then medical practice might be transformed to prioritize patience and caution over speedy, irrevocable interventions.

Such a change would be less radical than it may appear, however. It would preserve the principle that work is the right response to atypical sex anatomies. Holmes has complained that the terminology of disorder means that "*not* managing the child never enters into the logic of the diagnosis"; rather, treatment guidelines such as the policy statement simply alter the form of medical work "from immediate surgical intervention to (potentially) life-long psychological/psychiatric management."[66] Like Holmes, I think that if surgery were deferred or substituted by psychological support, then work would still be undertaken. But going beyond Holmes's argument, I want to draw attention to the diagnostic tests that precede decisions about treatment. As we have seen, such tests require specialized effort. To test a patient is to do work, irrespective of whether the test results may lead to a decision against early surgery. On the basis of their child's diagnosis, parents could decline all surgical options, but in so doing they would remain reliant upon the work of testing—on somebody else doing something in response to their child's body. Similarly, if patient support-group representatives became full "members of the care team," as two lead authors of the policy statement have suggested, they too would be working.[67] Tasks for support-group representatives proposed in official guidelines include helping patients and their families to understand the "condition" at hand, supporting their search for suitable medical care, and assisting them in recognizing "the reasons for medical therapy."[68] These tasks are focused on managing the knowledge of families and patients. I think, however, that by carrying out such specialized activities, patient support would be turned into a discipline like any other, characterized by a certain type of work. The work would be fundamentally conservative. Providing expert labor in knowledge management, support-group representatives in care teams would embody the expectation that work should be done instead of contesting it.

In this section, I have identified two key oppositions that organize the debate over the transformative power of the DSD terminology and its associated treatment guidelines. The first opposition is between individual and universal decisions about patient management. The second is between work and nonwork. As I have shown, existing arguments by several commentators proceed by showing that one side of each opposing pair eclipses its respective counterpart and thereby distorts the terms of the debate—for example, that individualized treatments obscure universal principles such as consent and that surgical work trivializes alternatives as if they are not work. In my view, all such arguments are incomplete. I argue instead that the whole opposition between the individual and the universal masks the fact that there is something else at play, something that is neither individual nor universal, but structural. I am referring to the structural explanation for the opposition between work and nonwork, which cannot be revealed by trying to decide whether

188 ‿ WAS INTERSEX REAL?

work should be done on either an individual or a universal basis. The name for this structure is the *mode of production*. In social theory, any society's mode of production determines which activities count as work—those that are productive—and therefore determines also what is meant by nonwork.[69] We remain uncritical of the prevailing mode of production if we focus on choosing between individual and universal approaches to work. Likewise, the question with which I opened this section— Should work be done at all?—is locked within the mode of production, for it is dependent on the structural separation of work from nonwork. By structuring work and nonwork in opposition, the prevailing mode of production forecloses the idea of doing anything in response to atypical sex characteristics that might be neither work nor nonwork. So the final challenge that I want to tackle in this chapter is whether something altogether different may be possible.

OUT OF TIME

Among doctors, a colloquialism for the misuse of hindsight to critique medical practices is the "retrospectoscope." It is a metaphorical tool for looking across time. Equipped with a retrospectoscope, anyone can be right. Five years before the conception of the DSD terminology, the pediatric endocrinologist Melvin Grumbach complained that some critics of twentieth-century intersex medicine "look through the retrospectoscope" to say, "My God! How did we do that?" According to Grumbach, such criticisms judge the past unfairly. "A lot has changed since then," Grumbach remarked; "we must learn from the advances that have been made rather than point fingers."[70] Since those comments, proponents of the DSD terminology have heralded the new terms and treatment guidelines as opportunities to change not only how medicine is practiced but also how it is critiqued. Coauthors of the 2006 policy statement have claimed that the term *DSD* has undone the idea of "intersex activism" and so has defused earlier criticisms that proceeded by "direct confrontation of the medical establishment."[71] In place of such finger pointing, they have urged for "constructive collaborations" between clinical practitioners and everybody else.[72] Reflecting on similar developments in women's healthcare, the cultural critic Victoria Grace has observed that the collapse of polarization between medicine and activism functions to "absorb and recapture any form of opposition." But, as Grace also notes, this is not because structural forces cease to exist—quite the opposite.[73] In the case of intersex, I think that the call for doctors and activists to be unanimously "constructive" remains governed by the mode of production. It implies that we can identify which activities constitute productive work, divide them from activities that are unproductive, and agree to pursue the former to the exclusion of the latter. In the collaborative era that medical policymakers envisage, the division between work and nonwork would heal the polarization between medicine and intersex activism. The retrospectoscope would be put aside. Everyone would converge onto being constructive.

Yet the call to be constructive rests on unstable foundations because of its reliance on an unambiguous definition of work. I am going to argue that no such definition is possible. Although the mode of production separates work from nonwork, it also hides the truth that not all medical work is productive and so cannot be distinguished conclusively from nonwork. To explain this point, consider that the aims of genital surgery include the avoidance of "stigmatization related to atypical anatomy," according to several coauthors of the policy statement.[74] Now, we might suppose that genital surgeries are unproductive only when they go wrong—on the occasions when they result in problems such as nerve damage, vaginal narrowing, obtrusive scarring, and urethral leakages. That is not my argument here. I think that genital surgeries are unproductive *even when they go right* because they fail to stop the stigmatization of genitalia that are cosmetically or functionally atypical. Moreover, such surgeries have the reverse effect than the one intended: for affected individuals who undergo surgery in childhood, our first experience of stigmatization is genital surgery itself.[75] Far from being unambiguously productive, therefore, surgery is an elaborately staged nonintervention—an act that takes no action against social stigma. This analysis raises the corresponding possibility that productive ways to address stigma may lie outside medical work. For instance, as an alternative to surgery, doctors and parents might use their authority to "truly destigmatize sexual variation by paying little attention to it," Sharon Preves suggests.[76] Responding with indifference to genitals that look unusual or function unexpectedly may not sound like work. Nevertheless, it may require a lot of effort by doctors and parents, and it may reduce stigma more than surgery does. Recognizing such indifference as potentially productive becomes feasible once we acknowledge the porosity of the distinction between work and nonwork.

Because the call for everyone to be constructive presupposes that work can be separated from nonwork, it requires us not to notice how productivity and unproductivity are entwined in medical practice. So even though medicine is habitually unproductive in destigmatizing atypical genitalia, it is structured in opposition to nonwork as though it were unequivocally productive. This is illustrated by remarks from the pediatricians Peter Lee and Christopher Houk, who were among the lead authors of both the original and follow-up policy statements. In a paper published in the years between the two statements, Lee and Houk appealed for patient-advocacy groups to unite with health professionals in pursuing "the singular goal of improving patient outcomes."[77] Their choice of words takes for granted that unalloyed work is possible and implies that medical practices have a readily identifiable "singular goal." I think this is a mischaracterization because, as I have argued throughout this book, the medical management of genital atypicality has never been a coherent enterprise. Holmes has likewise pointed out that genital surgeries in childhood neither "restore any clear function that is a universal and expected human trait" nor enhance the body.[78] These interventions do not make normal genitalia out of atypical genitalia: they make postsurgical genitalia, which are still atypical because most people in the world do not undergo genital surgery. The beneficiaries of such interventions are hazy, too; as I argued in chapter 3, early surgeries may be "proxy treatments of parental anxiety," in Holmes's phrasing, rather than actions taken to benefit affected children.[79] It is therefore questionable how far the medical management of atypical genitalia has ever been focused on patient outcomes, contrary to what Lee and Houk say. In this respect, the collaborations between medics and activists envisaged by proponents of the DSD terminology ask us to overlook the ambivalence of medical practices. Being "constructive" entails seeing genital surgery as if it were productive all along and seeing postsurgical genitalia as if they were normal.

Further, the structural opposition between medical practices and nonwork means that criticisms of medicine seem to be criticisms of work, and so they appear unfair. Lee and Houk call such criticisms "confrontational," juxtaposing them to the "constructive approach" that they favor. To demonstrate what they mean by "confrontational methods in attempts to rectify treatments," they cite occasions on which patient-advocacy groups have "demanded apologies from institutions and physicians who cared for children with DSD in the past." I think their comments reveal a core inconsistency in the view that the DSD terminology and guidelines are a break from earlier medical practices. On the one hand, Lee and Houk describe contemporary medicine as the best yet—"more humanistic" than before and free from "previous misconceptions" on fundamental points such as gender development, the importance of genital tactility, and the preservation of fertility. On the other hand, they rebuke some contemporary advocacy groups for calling on doctors to apologize to patients who were treated according to those very misconceptions, a call that Lee and Houk admonish as scapegoating. In short, they claim simultaneously that medical practices have improved and that previous practices are above criticism. Trying to reconcile this inconsistency, Lee and Houk assert that former patients have misremembered the treatments they received. They state that false memories, not medical treatments, are the source of "chronic resentment" among patients, which can "impede lifelong adjustment."[80] The authors thereby switch the stakes of the argument from misperceptions held by clinicians in the past to misperceptions of the past by patients. I consider this transposition a sleight of hand because medical interventions have traditionally been scheduled in early childhood specifically to make them difficult to comprehend. The inability to understand treatment is one of its intentionally traumatizing effects, as I discussed in chapter 2.[81] So instead of demonstrating that it is unfair for advocacy groups to seek apologies for former patients, the memory problems invoked by Lee and Houk are really an illustration of why previous treatments deserve criticism.

In this section, I have been exploring how the mode of production, despite its instability, operates to limit critique. Rather than illuminating how medicine itself may not be constructive, the appeal for everybody to be constructive has the reverse effect: it categorizes the scrutiny of unproductive medical practices as a failure to behave constructively. This is a centrally important point in my argument. The mode of production shuts down the possibility that critique could have a purpose. It means that critique cannot initiate change under the prevailing mode of production. The cultural theorist Fredric Jameson has written that every mode of production "produces a temporality that is specific to it."[82] By this, Jameson means that the structural separation between work and nonwork defines our experience of the relationship between past, present, and future. Behind the claim that medical interventions are needed to alleviate social stigma in the present lies the perception that changing society is impossible and that it is easier to imagine surgical and hormonal interventions on children than to imagine a more accommodating social world in the future. Intertwined with this perception is the sense that medical practices, unlike society, have already changed for the better through "the advances that have been made" in the past, as Grumbach put it. The result is a failure to imagine a future that contains anything besides more medical work—a simple reiteration of the present mode of production. This reiteration is typified by comments made by the pediatric urologist Mark Woodward. In the year of the follow-up policy statement, 2016, Woodward rejected calls to defer genital surgery from infancy to adolescence on the grounds that deferral would prevent surgeons from gaining the experience necessary to perform surgery when patients are older.[83] In this circuitous temporality, work is necessary now so that it can be done in the future, even though work should not be postponed to the future, but done now. Immobilized between medical advances that have already happened and social tolerance that will never arrive, critique has no role within this perpetual present of medical work.

The retrospectoscope, then, is not the only tool for looking across time. The mode of production also organizes how we see medical practices in the past, present, and future. So the alternative to the retrospectoscope is not simple neutrality. More than being the backdrop to the DSD terminology and treatment guidelines, the mode of production is also the structure through which we perceive their effects over time. In the light of this analysis, it may seem that the only conceivable outcome from the introduction of the DSD terminology is interminable medicalization—no change, only continuity. However, such a conclusion would miss something vitally important. In concluding this book, I want to show that there is another way; although the separation between work and nonwork is structural, that does not make it entirely rigid. I have argued that the mode of production is unstable, which leaves open the possibility of a different activity that is neither work nor nonwork. I am referring to *the attempt to define work*. As we have seen, this attempt at definition fails. It cannot succeed because work and nonwork cannot be cleaved. Yet the failure is key. I do not think it is an accident that might be overcome by devising a better definition of work; instead, it is reflective of the instability in the mode of production. In other words, it is a failure that tells the truth. Through failing, the attempt to define work constitutes a type of activity that is not productive but is not simply unproductive, either, for it reveals the untruth of the mode of production. Turning sideways from the customary opposition between doing something and doing nothing, this act of failure cannot be subsumed by the structural categorization of productive labor within current societal arrangements. It shows that the mode of production does not govern everything that can happen—that its temporality is not quite a closed circuit after all. So in response to atypical sex anatomies, we do not have to select between doing something and doing nothing. We can do something else. We can think.

Afterword

RESISTING MEDICAL NECESSITY

While I was writing this book, the COVID-19 pandemic of the early 2020s happened. A dark irony of the pandemic was that just as everyday life for many of us became unremittingly medicalized, the intense demand on medical providers prompted the quiet deferral of some intersex surgeries—a tacit recognition by clinicians that many such procedures were never really necessary.[1] In this afterword, I want to reflect on the fact that the border between necessary and unnecessary interventions acts as a natural limit to the scope of intersex criticism, including my own. It demarcates a rump of medical treatments, whether hormonal or surgical, that are beyond critique because of their presumed necessity. This is exemplified by the contrast between hormone-replacement therapy for life-threatening chemical deficiencies that occur when an intersex body makes testosterone in lieu of other chemicals, versus surgery to change the appearance of a clitoris that has been enlarged by the resulting testosterone. The former is necessary; the latter is unnecessary. Not only is the latter intervention decidedly cosmetic, but it also does nothing to solve the chemical problem, and the stress of surgery in fact aggravates the chemical deficiency.[2]

Also in the time it took to write this book, five countries introduced national legislation to curtail medical interventions for intersex during childhood—Germany, Greece, Iceland, Malta, and Portugal.[3] These laws are astounding developments and victories for intersex activism. All the new laws draw a distinction between medical interventions that are unnecessary in childhood, which they ban, and other medical interventions that are necessary, which they permit subject to parental consent. None of the laws names specific procedures in either category, surgical or otherwise. They instead categorize the unnecessary interventions as those that are driven by social or cosmetic concerns and the necessary interventions as those that are motivated by children's health. In this respect, the legal reforms echo long-running efforts by critics of intersex medicine to distinguish between necessary and unnecessary interventions with a view to focusing critiques on the latter.[4] Unfortunately, however, there is little sign that the legal reforms are truly changing medical practices, even in Malta, where such legislation has been in place the longest.[5]

Although the difference between necessary and unnecessary medical interventions is manifestly clear in some situations, that is not always the case. For example, surgery that seeks to enable a boy to urinate in a standing position addresses urinary function, but the functionality at stake is socially determined—it is more usual for boys and men to stand while urinating in the United States than in, say, Germany.[6] Likewise, the necessity of some surgeries may be driven by complications from earlier surgeries. For instance, a urethral stricture that blocks urination may require urgent remediation, but its urgency is a side effect of medicalization rather than a preexisting bodily need. Moreover, doctors who extol the narrative of continuous medical progress often advocate combining multiple surgical procedures into a single intervention during childhood on the basis that this combination constitutes the most efficient form of surgery.[7] Such interventions blur together functional and cosmetic changes to children's bodies, making it difficult to specify the extent to which they are necessary or unnecessary.[8] They also make it ever more confusing for parents to understand exactly what they are choosing when they choose surgery for their children.

In response to such uncertainty, some critics argue that the way forward would be for lawmakers and policymakers to be more prescriptive about which procedures count as necessary.[9] While such a move would provide temporary clarity, I suspect that the category of "medical necessity" will creep outward as new types of intervention become technically possible: Innovations in medical technology will continue to unsettle the borders between what seems possible, what feels necessary, and what is actually needed. More fundamentally, the focus on stopping medically unnecessary interventions means that critics of medicine will always be beholden to medical authority to establish the boundaries of necessity. This dependency is caused by the professionalization of healthcare in late-modern societies. It would appear, then, that truly demedicalizing intersex is an unfeasible goal. As a matter of fact, we could say that the aim of stopping *unnecessary* medical interventions is at odds with the aim of complete demedicalization, even though at a glance they seem like two ways of expressing the same objective.

Meanwhile, for doctors and parents who continue to advocate the conventional medical management of intersex, the figure of the intersex adult who was never surgically normalized in childhood is both inconceivable and threatening. This is a figure on whose stigmatization medicine depends to justify early genital surgeries. To describe oneself as proud, joyful, and healthy without medically unnecessary surgeries is an existential danger to intersex medicine. As the activist Nthabiseng Mokoena has declared, "To the doctor that told my mother that surgery is necessary when I was an infant, . . . here I am right now, still no surgery, still not sick, still healthy, still bouncy, still happy, still awesome."[10] Indeed, since John Money's gender theory that originally underpinned intersex medical management has been discredited, and as legal reforms spread, some doctors are grasping for evidence by any measure that intersex adults who did not receive normalizing surgery must have terrible lives.[11] Nevertheless, while intersex medicine is stalked by the figure of the adult who never received the socially and cosmetically driven interventions that critics of medical treatment call unnecessary, I think intersex criticism is haunted by an altogether different figure.

We have collectively invested a great deal of energy and optimism in the figure of the child who undergoes strictly medically necessary interventions alone.[12] That child represents the great hope of intersex activism—a child who was never normalized and who is free to choose or eschew surgeries later as they please. But I am not referring to that child here. In closing this book, I suggest there is another figure in the shadows whose presence is key to holding medicine to account: the intersex individual who has not undergone even medically necessary interventions. We might call this figure "disabled." This radically demedicalized, disabled figure challenges critics of medicine to remain vigilant over the scope of medical necessity even as we invoke that category to propel vital changes in medical practice.[13] They bring us face to face with our assumptions about the circumstances in which we think medical interventions would be obvious. Beyond unnecessary and necessary interventions alike, beyond both medicine and criticism, this twilight figure demands that critics of medicalization never stop questioning how we define the parameters of a livable life.

ACKNOWLEDGMENTS

For helpful conversations and sharing information, I thank Neil Badmington, Sarah Creighton, Leah DeVun, Lisa Downing, Victoria Grace, Laura Gregory, Nadine Gulde, Peter Hegarty, and Lih-Mei Liao. In addition, I thank Wendy Lochner, the team, and readers at Columbia University Press for their thoughtful feedback that improved this book. The editors and readers at *differences* and *GLQ* also made valuable suggestions regarding earlier versions of chapters 1 and 4, respectively.

An earlier version of chapter 1 appeared as "The Injured World: Intersex and the Phenomenology of Feeling," *differences: A Journal of Feminist Cultural Studies* 23, no. 2 (2012): 20–41, © copyright 2012, Brown University and *differences: A Journal of Feminist Cultural Studies*. All rights reserved. Republished by permission of the publisher.

An earlier version of chapter 4 appeared as "What Can Queer Theory Do for Intersex?," *GLQ: A Journal of Lesbian and Gay Studies* 15, no. 2 (2009): 285–312, © copyright 2009, Duke University Press. All rights reserved. Republished by permission of the publisher.

NOTES

INTRODUCTION: DECONSTRUCTING INTERSEX MEDICINE

1. M. Morgan Holmes, *Intersex: A Perilous Difference* (Susquehanna University Press, 2008), 70.

2. David Andrew Griffiths, "Shifting Syndromes: Sex Chromosome Variations and Intersex Classifications," *Social Studies of Science* 48, no. 1 (2018): 128–29; Amanda Lock Swarr, *Envisioning African Intersex: Challenging Colonial and Racist Legacies in South African Medicine* (Duke University Press, 2023), 49–61.

3. Andreas Kyriakou et al., "Current Models of Care for Disorders of Sex Development: Results from an International Survey of Specialist Centres," *Orphanet Journal of Rare Diseases* 11 (2016): art. 155, https://doi.org/10.1186/s13023-016-0534-8.

4. Isabelle Vidal et al., "Surgical Options in Disorders of Sex Development (DSD) with Ambiguous Genitalia," *Best Practice & Research Clinical Endocrinology & Metabolism* 24, no. 2 (2010): 311–24. The extent to which sterilizations (gonadectomies) are intended to avoid perceived sexual ambiguity or to mitigate future cancer risks is particularly contentious. The latter risks vary widely between types of intersex, and there is no consensus on the level of risk that would warrant gonadectomy rather than regular screening. See Lih-Mei Liao, *Variations in Sex Development: Medicine, Culture, and Psychological Practice* (Cambridge University Press, 2023), 49.

5. Zoltan Hrabovszky and John M. Hutson, "Surgical Treatment of Intersex Abnormalities: A Review," *Surgery* 131, no. 1 (2002): 101.

6. Berenice Bilharinho Mendonca et al., "46,XY Disorders of Sex Development (DSD)," *Clinical Endocrinology* 70, no. 2 (2009): 183–84.

7. John Money, "Hermaphroditism, Gender, and Precocity in Hyperadrenocorticism: Psychologic Findings," *Bulletin of the Johns Hopkins Hospital* 96, no. 6 (1955): 257.

8. Sean Saifa Wall and Pidgeon Pagonis, "Creating Intersex Justice: Interview with Sean Saifa Wall and Pidgeon Pagonis of the Intersex Justice Project," interview by David A. Rubin et al., *Transgender Studies Quarterly* 9, no. 2 (2022): 193; Anne Tamar-Mattis, "Medical Treatment of People with Intersex Conditions as Torture and Cruel, Inhuman, or Degrading Treatment or Punishment," in *Torture in Healthcare Settings: Reflections on the Special Rapporteur on Torture's 2013 Thematic Report*, ed. Center for Human Rights and Humanitarian Law (American University, 2014), 102.

9. On hormonal treatments, see Peter A. Lee, Anna Nordenström, et al., "Global Disorders of Sex Development Update Since 2006: Perceptions, Approach, and Care," *Hormone Research in Paediatrics* 85, no. 3 (2016): 172; on vaginal dilations, see Amanda Wee et al., "Creation and Maintenance of Neo-Vagina with the Use of Vaginal Dilators as First Line Treatment: Results from a Quaternary Paediatric and Adolescent Gynaecology Service in Australia," *Australian and New Zealand Journal of Obstetrics and Gynaecology* 62, no. 3 (2022): 439–44; on urethral dilations, see Tong Shi et al., "One-Stage Tubularized Urethroplasty Using the Free Inner Plate of the Foreskin in the Treatment of Proximal Hypospadias," *BMC Pediatrics* 22 (2022): art. 393, https://doi.org /10.1186/s12887-022-03464-2, 3; on follow-up surgeries, see Naomi S. Crouch and Sarah M. Creighton, "Long-Term Functional Outcomes of Female Genital Reconstruction in Childhood," *BJU International* 100, no. 2 (2007): 404.

10. Paula Sandrine Machado et al., "Follow-up of Psychological Outcomes of Interventions in Patients Diagnosed with Disorders of Sexual Development: A Systematic Review," *Journal of Health Psychology* 21, no. 10 (2016): 2204–5.

11. Daniel M. Weber et al., "The Pediatric Penile Perception Score: An Instrument for Patient Self-Assessment and Surgeon Evaluation After Hypospadias Repair," *Journal of Urology* 180, no. 3 (2008): 1080; Mario Lima et al., "Vaginal Replacement in the Pediatric Age Group: A 34-Year Experience of Intestinal Vaginoplasty in Children and Young Girls," *Journal of Pediatric Surgery* 45, no. 10 (2010): 2087–91; A. Farkas et al.,"1-Stage Feminizing Genitoplasty: 8 Years of Experience with 49 Cases," *Journal of Urology* 165, no. 6 (2001): 2341–46.

12. Alice Domurat Dreger, "'Ambiguous Sex'—or Ambivalent Medicine? Ethical Issues in the Treatment of Intersexuality," *Hastings Center Report* 28, no. 3 (1998): 32.

13. Robert A. Crouch, "Betwixt and Between: The Past and Future of Intersexuality," in *Intersex in the Age of Ethics*, ed. Alice Domurat Dreger (University Publishing Group, 1999), 32–34.

14. Renata Ziemińska, "Toward a Nonbinary Model of Gender/Sex Traits," *Hypatia* 37, no. 2 (2022): 418.

15. Suzanne J. Kessler, *Lessons from the Intersexed* (Rutgers University Press, 1998), 30–32.

16. Cheryl Chase, "Affronting Reason," in *Looking Queer: Body Image and Identity in Lesbian, Bisexual, Gay, and Transgender Communities*, ed. Dawn Atkins (Harrington Park, 1998), 208.

17. Morgan Carpenter, "The Human Rights of Intersex People: Addressing Harmful Practices and Rhetoric of Change," *Reproductive Health Matters* 24, no. 47 (2016): 77–78.

18. Iain Morland, "Gender, Genitals, and the Meaning of Being Human," in Lisa Downing et al., *Fuckology: Critical Essays on John Money's Diagnostic Concepts* (University of Chicago Press, 2015), 69–98.

19. Katrina Karkazis, *Fixing Sex: Intersex, Medical Authority, and Lived Experience* (Duke University Press, 2008), 249.

20. Claire Nihoul-Fékété, "How to Deal with Congenital Disorders of Sex Development in 2008 (DSD)," *European Journal of Pediatric Surgery* 18, no. 6 (2008): 366; Caroline Sanders et al., "Parents' Narratives About Their Experiences of Their Child's Reconstructive Genital Surgeries for Ambiguous Genitalia," *Journal of Clinical Nursing* 17, no. 23 (2007): 3192.

21. Griffiths, "Shifting Syndromes," 143.

22. Hida Viloria, "Promoting Health and Social Progress by Accepting and Depathologizing Benign Intersex Traits," *Narrative Inquiry in Bioethics* 5, no. 2 (2015): 116–17.

23. For example, on medical practices in Aotearoa/New Zealand, the United Kingdom, and the United States, respectively, see Claire Breen and Katrina Roen, "The Rights of Intersex Children in Aotearoa New Zealand," *International Journal of Children's Rights* 31, no. 3 (2023): 537–43; Surya Monro et al., *Intersex, Variations of Sex Characteristics, and DSD: The Need for Change* (University of Huddersfield, 2017), 11–15; and Human Rights Watch, *"I Want to Be Like Nature Made Me": Medically Unnecessary Surgeries on Intersex Children in the US* (Human Rights Watch, 2017), 48–49.

24. Sonia R. Grover et al., "Introduction: Changing Landscapes," in *Disorders\Differences of Sex Development: An Integrated Approach to Management*, 2nd ed., ed. John M. Hutson et al. (Springer Nature Singapore, 2020), 9–10.

25. Martine Cools et al., "Caring for Individuals with a Difference of Sex Development (DSD): A Consensus Statement," *Nature Reviews Endocrinology* 14, no. 7 (2018): 426.

26. Fae Garland and Mitchell Travis, "Temporal Bodies: Emergencies, Emergence, and Intersex Embodiment," in *A Jurisprudence of the Body*, ed. Chris Dietz et al. (Palgrave Macmillan, 2020), 131.

27. Theodor W. Adorno, *Prisms* (1955), trans. Samuel Weber and Shierry Weber (Neville Spearman, 1967), 32.

28. Key monographs in the critical study of intersex medicine are: From anthropology, Karkazis, *Fixing Sex*. From gender studies, Lena Eckert, *Intersexualization: The Clinic and the Colony* (Routledge, 2017); and David A. Rubin, *Intersex Matters: Biomedical Embodiment, Gender Regulation, and Transnational Activism* (State University of New York Press, 2017). From law, Julie A. Greenberg, *Intersexuality and the Law: Why Sex Matters* (New York University Press, 2012); and Fae Garland and Mitchell Travis, *Intersex Embodiment: Legal Frameworks Beyond Identity and Disorder* (Bristol University Press, 2023). From philosophy, Ellen K. Feder, *Making Sense of Intersex: Changing Ethical Perspectives in Biomedicine* (Indiana University Press, 2014). From psychology, Kessler, *Lessons from the Intersexed*; and Liao, *Variations in Sex Development*.

From sociology, Sharon E. Preves, *Intersex and Identity: The Contested Self* (Rutgers University Press, 2003); and Georgiann Davis, *Contesting Intersex: The Dubious Diagnosis* (New York University Press, 2015). Key interdisciplinary monographs that draw on fields such as feminist science studies, media studies, and disability studies are Holmes, *Intersex*; Hil Malatino (as Hilary Malatino), *Queer Embodiment: Monstrosity, Medical Violence, and Intersex Experience* (University of Nebraska Press, 2019); Celeste E. Orr, *Cripping Intersex* (UBC Press, 2022); and Swarr, *Envisioning African Intersex*. On the historical development of intersex medicine, key monographs are Alice Domurat Dreger, *Hermaphrodites and the Medical Invention of Sex* (Harvard University Press, 1998); Geertje Mak, *Doubting Sex: Inscriptions, Bodies, and Selves in Nineteenth-Century Hermaphrodite Case Histories* (Manchester University Press, 2012); and Elizabeth Reis, *Bodies in Doubt: An American History of Intersex*, 2nd ed. (Johns Hopkins University Press, 2021). Key autobiographical books are Thea Hillman, *Intersex (for Lack of a Better Word)* (Manic D Press, 2008); Hida Viloria, *Born Both: An Intersex Life* (Hachette, 2017); Eric Lohman and Stephani Lohman, *Raising Rosie: Our Story of Parenting an Intersex Child* (Jessica Kingsley, 2018); and Kimberly M. Zieselman, *XOXY: A Memoir* (Jessica Kingsley, 2020).

29. Downing et al., *Fuckology*.

30. For example, just like Money, the Endocrine Society professional association claims that sex reassignment is possible in early childhood because young children have not yet achieved "consistent self-labeling by gender." See Phyllis W. Speiser et al., "Congenital Adrenal Hyperplasia due to Steroid 21-Hydroxylase Deficiency: An Endocrine Society Clinical Practice Guideline," *Journal of Clinical Endocrinology and Metabolism* 103, no. 11 (2018): 4070; and John Money, *The Psychologic Study of Man* (Charles C. Thomas, 1957), 51.

31. Arthur W. Frank, *The Wounded Storyteller: Body, Illness, and Ethics* (University of Chicago Press, 1995), 144.

32. Limor Meoded Danon argues that the intersex body is a kind of archive. See Meoded Danon, "Temporal Sociomedical Approaches to Intersex* Bodies," *History and Philosophy of the Life Sciences* 44, no. 2 (2022): art. 28, https://doi.org/10.1007/s40656-022-00511-0, 3–4.

33. The most notorious example of how sex testing leads to bodily interventions is Patrick Fénichel et al., "Molecular Diagnosis of 5α-Reductase Deficiency in 4 Elite Young Female Athletes Through Hormonal Screening for Hyperandrogenism," *Journal of Clinical Endocrinology and Metabolism* 98, no. 6 (2013): e1055–59. The authors, based in France and Monaco, performed "a partial clitoridectomy with a bilateral gonadectomy" on four women "from rural or mountainous regions of developing countries," after which the women were "allowed . . . to continue competing in the female category" (e1057, e1056).

34. On this issue, see, for example, Orr, *Cripping Intersex*, 144–81; Rubin, *Intersex Matters*, 121–40; and Swarr, *Envisioning African Intersex*, 102–31.

35. For example, Intersex Society of North America, "Why Doesn't ISNA Want to Eradicate Gender?," 2006, https://www.isna.org/faq/not _eradicating_gender, para. 6 of 7; Viloria, *Born Both*, 111.

36. Kessler, *Lessons from the Intersexed*, 132; Rubin, *Intersex Matters*, 21–48.

37. On the historical connection and Money's work, see Jules Gill-Peterson (as Julian Gill-Peterson), *Histories of the Transgender Child* (University of Minnesota Press, 2018), 126–27.

38. Alice Domurat Dreger and April M. Herndon, "Progress and Politics in the Intersex Rights Movement: Feminist Theory in Action," *GLQ* 15, no. 2 (2009): 212–13; Michelle Wolff et al., "The Intersex Issue: An Introduction," *Transgender Studies Quarterly* 9, no. 2 (2022): 148–51.

39. Heino F. L. Meyer-Bahlburg, "The Timing of Genital Surgery in Somatic Intersexuality: Surveys of Patients' Preferences," *Hormone Research in Paediatrics* 95, no. 1 (2022): 17.

40. For an example of my work on transgender and intersex, see Iain Morland, "Intersex Surgery Between the Gaze and the Subject," *Transgender Studies Quarterly* 9, no. 2 (2022): 168–69.

41. Liao, *Variations in Sex Development*, 62–71, esp. 65.

42. Relatedly, some authors now use names that are different from those under which they published the sources that I cite. In the body of this book, I have used everybody's current names to the best of my knowledge. In the notes and bibliography, I have added

the names under which sources were published to help readers find them.

43. Liao, *Variations in Sex Development*, 104.

1. THE INJURED WORLD

1. For further discussion of this ambivalent sentiment, see Line Merete Mediå et al., "'It Was Supposed to Be a Secret': A Study of Disclosure and Stigma as Experienced by Adults with Differences of Sex Development," *Health Psychology and Behavioral Medicine* 10, no. 1 (2022): 589.

2. Kathleen Lennon, "Making Life Livable: Transsexuality and Bodily Transformation," *Radical Philosophy*, no. 140 (2006): 28.

3. Rosalyn Diprose, *The Bodies of Women: Ethics, Embodiment, and Sexual Difference* (Routledge, 1994), 104.

4. Alice Domurat Dreger, "Jarring Bodies: Thoughts on the Display of Unusual Anatomies," *Perspectives in Biology and Medicine* 43, no. 2 (2000): 171.

5. Karkazis, *Fixing Sex*, 246–47.

6. This striking metaphor comes from D. T. Wilcox and P. G. Ransley, "Medicolegal Aspects of Hypospadias," *BJU International* 86, no. 3 (2000): 329.

7. Readers who are familiar with the version of this chapter that appeared in the journal *differences* may notice that there I stated that I had fourteen surgeries, not fifteen. When I reread my medical records and pieced together the sequence of events from letters between clinicians, I discovered an additional procedure that took place in childhood. It is a good example of how treatment distorts autobiographical understanding. See Iain Morland, "The Injured World: Intersex and the Phenomenology of Feeling," *differences: A Journal of Feminist Cultural Studies* 23, no. 2 (2012): 22.

8. Alice Domurat Dreger, "Intersex and Human Rights: The Long View," in *Ethics and Intersex*, ed. Sharon E. Sytsma (Springer, 2006), 80, emphasis in original.

9. Anne Fausto-Sterling, *Myths of Gender: Biological Theories About Women and Men* (Basic, 1985), 133–41; Suzanne J. Kessler, "The Medical

Construction of Gender: Case Management of Intersexed Infants,"
Signs 16, no. 1 (1990): 3–26; Cheryl Chase, "Intersexual Rights" (letter),
Sciences 33, no. 4 (1993): 3; M. Morgan Holmes, "Queer Cut Bodies:
Intersexuality and Homophobia in Medical Practice," University of
Southern California, 1995, https://web.archive.org/web/20060703155923
/http://www.usc.edu/libraries/archives/queerfrontiers/queer/papers
/holmes.long.html; Dreger, *Hermaphrodites*.

10. Justine Marut Schober, "A Surgeon's Response to the Intersex Controversy," in *Intersex in the Age of Ethics*, ed. Dreger, 161–68; Sarah M.
Creighton, "Surgery for Intersex," *Journal of the Royal Society of Medicine* 94, no. 5 (2001): 218–20; William G. Reiner, "Assignment of Sex
in Neonates with Ambiguous Genitalia," *Current Opinion in Pediatrics* 11, no. 4 (1999): 363–65.

11. For example, Alice Domurat Dreger, "A History of Intersex: From the
Age of Gonads to the Age of Consent," in *Intersex in the Age of Ethics*,
ed. Dreger, 16–17.

12. Chase, "Intersexual Rights," 3.

13. Emily Grabham, "Bodily Integrity and the Surgical Management of
Intersex," *Body & Society* 18, no. 2 (2012): 21.

14. Esther Morris, "The Self I Will Never Know," *New Internationalist*,
January–February 2004, 25.

15. Cheryl Chase, "What Is the Agenda of the Intersex Patient Advocacy
Movement?," *Endocrinologist* 13, no. 3 (2003): 240.

16. Dreger, *Hermaphrodites*, 167–201.

17. Dreger, *Hermaphrodites*, 168–70; Eli Nevada and Cheryl Chase, "Natural Allies," *Hermaphrodites with Attitude*, Summer 1995, 1.

18. Milton Diamond, "A Critical Evaluation of the Ontogeny of Human
Sexual Behavior," *Quarterly Review of Biology* 40, no. 2 (1965): 147–75.

19. Kessler, *Lessons from the Intersexed*, 132.

20. See Orr, *Cripping Intersex*, 14–15, on the potential and limitations of
the social model of disability.

21. Sandra Lipsitz Bem, "Dismantling Gender Polarization and Compulsory Heterosexuality: Should We Turn the Volume Down or Up?"
Journal of Sex Research 32, no. 4 (1995): 329–30.

22. Chase, "Affronting Reason," 214, emphasis in original.

23. Limor Meoded Danon, "The Body/Secret Dynamic: Life Experiences of Intersexed People in Israel," *SAGE Open* 5, no. 2 (2015), https://doi .org/10.1177/2158244015580370, 11.

24. Jorge Daaboul and Joel Frader, "Ethics and the Management of the Patient with Intersex: A Middle Way," *Journal of Pediatric Endocrinology and Metabolism* 14, no. 9 (2001): 1577.

25. Anne Fausto-Sterling, "The Five Sexes: Why Male and Female Are Not Enough," *Sciences* 33, no. 2 (1993): 21.

26. For example, Martina Jürgensen et al., "'Any Decision Is Better Than None': Decision-Making About Sex of Rearing for Siblings with 17β-Hydroxysteroid-Dehydrogenase-3 Deficiency," *Archives of Sexual Behavior* 35, no. 3 (2006): 364.

27. Laura Inter (pseud.), "Finding My Compass," trans. Leslie Jaye, *Narrative Inquiry in Bioethics* 5, no. 2 (2015): 97.

28. Elaine Scarry, *The Body in Pain: The Making and Unmaking of the World* (Oxford University Press, 1985), 3–4.

29. In other words, identities are normative, not descriptive. See K. Anthony Appiah, "Identity, Authenticity, Survival: Multicultural Societies and Social Reproduction," in *Multiculturalism: Examining the Politics of Recognition*, ed. Amy Gutmann (Princeton University Press, 1994), 149–63. I explore the implications of a normative theory of identity further in "Why Five Sexes Are Not Enough," in *The Ashgate Research Companion to Queer Theory*, ed. Noreen Giffney and Michael O'Rourke (Ashgate, 2009), 33–47.

30. Viloria, *Born Both*, 256.

31. A way forward may be to establish "sex characteristics" as a "protected category that can only be modified with the individual's consent," in the words of Daniela Crocetti, Adeline Berry, and Surya Monro. See Crocetti, Berry, et al., "Navigating the Complexities of Adult Healthcare for Individuals with Variations of Sex Characteristics: From Paediatric Emergencies to a Sense of Abandonment," *Culture, Health, & Sexuality* 26, no. 3 (2024): 334.

32. Cheryl Chase quoted in Sarah Horowitz, "The Middle Sex," *San Francisco Weekly*, February 1, 1995. Hida Viloria also makes this comparison in a slightly different way in *Born Both*, 194.

33. I am grateful to an anonymous reader whose comments on my manu-
script sharpened my thinking about the nature of this comparison. As
Janet E. Halley notes, "'Like race' arguments are so intrinsically woven
into American discourses of equal justice that they can never be entirely
foregone," but rather than comparing "the traits of subordinated
groups," it is preferable to compare "the dynamics of subordination."
See Halley, "'Like Race' Arguments," in *What's Left of Theory? New
Work on the Politics of Literary Theory*, ed. Judith Butler et al. (Routledge, 2000), 46, 51.

34. Trina Grillo and Stephanie M. Wildman, "Obscuring the Importance
of Race: The Implication of Making Comparisons Between Racism
and Sexism (or Other -Isms)," *Duke Law Journal*, no. 2 (1991): 404–5.

35. Morland, "Gender, Genitals, and the Meaning of Being Human,"
84–90.

36. Zine Magubane, "Spectacles and Scholarship: Caster Semenya, Intersex Studies, and the Problem of Race in Feminist Theory," *Signs* 39,
no. 3 (2014): 781.

37. Lauren Berlant, "The Subject of True Feeling: Pain, Privacy, and Politics," in *Cultural Pluralism, Identity Politics, and the Law*, ed. Austin
Sarat and Thomas R. Kearns (University of Michigan Press, 1999), 58.
In a response to the earlier published version of the present chapter,
David A. Rubin highlighted the feeling of exhaustion among intersex
rights campaigners. Whereas Berlant's original formulation centered
on the inaction arising from mistaking good feelings for justice, the
risk of inaction from exhaustion shows how injustice can generate
feelings that wear down those who seek to oppose it. See Rubin,
"Anger, Aggression, Attitude: Intersex Rage as Biopolitical Protest,"
Signs 46, no. 4 (2021): 1006–7.

38. Iain Morland, "Between Critique and Reform: Ways of Reading the
Intersex Controversy," in *Critical Intersex*, ed. M. Morgan Holmes
(Ashgate, 2009), 208.

39. Chase, "What Is the Agenda of the Intersex Patient Advocacy Movement?," 242.

40. Arguably, some surgical procedures routinely undertaken for children
are at least partially cosmetic, such as cleft palate repairs. In an
argument against deferring all "gender-confirming" intersex genital

surgeries until patients are old enough to consent, Heino Meyer-Bahlburg has pointed out that early cleft palate surgeries are not ethically contentious. Meyer-Bahlburg suggests this shows that "ethical concerns" such as patient autonomy should not trigger the deferral of intersex childhood surgeries. However, as Anne Tamar-Mattis has countered, the scale of criticisms about childhood genital surgeries voiced by former patients distinguishes these interventions from cleft palate repairs. Even so, cleft palate surgeries do have some similarities to intersex surgeries, as Laura Hermer has noted, inasmuch as their results only approximate "normality," and they sometimes require multiple revisions. Yet this could be an argument to defer *both* cleft palate *and* intersex surgeries, contrary to what Meyer-Bahlburg and Tamar-Mattis say. See Heino Meyer-Bahlburg, "Misrepresentation of Evidence Favoring Early Normalizing Surgery for Atypical Sex Anatomies: Response to Baratz and Feder" (letter), *Archives of Sexual Behavior* 44, no. 7 (2015): 1765, 1767; Anne Tamar-Mattis, "Exceptions to the Rule: Curing the Law's Failure to Protect Intersex Infants," *Berkeley Journal of Gender, Law, and Justice* 21, no. 1 (2006): 71 n. 80; and Laura D. Hermer, "A Moratorium on Intersex Surgeries? Law, Science, Identity, and Bioethics at the Crossroads," *Cardozo Journal of Law and Gender* 13, no. 2 (2007): 271.

41. Melissa Hendricks, "Is It a Boy or a Girl?," *Johns Hopkins Magazine*, November 1993; John Money and Anke A. Ehrhardt, *Man and Woman, Boy and Girl: The Differentiation and Dimorphism of Gender Identity from Conception to Maturity* (Johns Hopkins University Press, 1972), 152.

42. For example, Kessler, *Lessons from the Intersexed*, 36.

43. Justine Marut Schober, "Feminization (Surgical Aspects)" (1998), in *Pediatric Surgery and Urology: Long-Term Outcomes*, 2nd ed., ed. Mark Stringer et al. (Cambridge University Press, 2006), 607.

44. Dreger and Herndon, "Progress and Politics in the Intersex Rights Movement," 212.

45. Dreger and Herndon, "Progress and Politics in the Intersex Rights Movement," 208.

46. Viloria, *Born Both*, 205.

47. Ellen K. Feder, "Imperatives of Normality: From 'Intersex' to 'Disorders of Sex Development,'" *GLQ* 15, no. 2 (2009): 240–41.

48. For example, Organisation Intersex International, "Alice Dreger: Disorders of Sex Development," 2007, https://web.archive.org/web/20111216120824/http://www.intersexualite.org/AliceDreger.html.

49. S. Faisal Ahmed, John C. Achermann, et al., "UK Guidance on the Initial Evaluation of an Infant or an Adolescent with a Suspected Disorder of Sex Development," *Clinical Endocrinology* 75, no. 1 (2011): 13–14.

50. On surgery remaining the typical approach to intersex, see Lina Michala et al., "Practice Changes in Childhood Surgery for Ambiguous Genitalia?," *Journal of Pediatric Urology* 10, no. 5 (2014): 934–40.

51. Maurice Merleau-Ponty, *The Visible and the Invisible* (1964), ed. Claude Lefort, trans. Alphonso Lingis (Northwestern University Press, 1968), 134.

52. Cary Gabriel Costello, "Understanding Intersex Relationship Issues," in *Expanding the Rainbow: Exploring the Relationships of Bi+, Polyamorous, Kinky, Ace, Intersex, and Trans People*, ed. Brandy L. Simula et al. (Brill, 2019), 241.

53. M. Morgan Holmes, "The Intersex Enchiridion: Naming and Knowledge," *Somatechnics* 1, no. 2 (2011): 398.

54. Iris Marion Young, "Throwing Like a Girl: A Phenomenology of Feminine Body Comportment, Motility, and Spatiality" (1980), in *Throwing Like a Girl and Other Essays in Feminist Philosophy and Social Theory* (Indiana University Press, 1990), 141–59.

55. Kristin Zeiler and Anette Wickström, "Why Do 'We' Perform Surgery on Newborn Intersexed Children? The Phenomenology of the Parental Experience of Having a Child with Intersex Anatomies," *Feminist Theory* 10, no. 3 (2009): 370.

56. Melissa L. Cull, "A Support Group's Perspective," *British Medical Journal* 330, no. 7487 (2005): 341.

57. Zeiler and Wickström, "Why Do 'We' Perform Surgery on Newborn Intersexed Children?," 371.

58. Young, "Throwing Like a Girl," 143.

59. Havi Carel, *Phenomenology of Illness* (Oxford University Press, 2016), 218–21.

60. Margrit Shildrick, *Leaky Bodies and Boundaries: Feminism, Postmodernism, and (Bio)Ethics* (Routledge, 1997); Margrit Shildrick, "Unreformed

Bodies: Normative Anxiety and the Denial of Pleasure," *Women's Studies* 34, nos. 3–4 (2005): 329. I discuss the conflation of touching and tactility more in chapter 4.

61. For example, M. Morgan Holmes, "Distracted Attentions: Intersexuality and Human Rights Protections," *Cardozo Journal of Law and Gender* 12, no. 1 (2005): 133.

62. Matthew Ratcliffe, *Feelings of Being: Phenomenology, Psychiatry, and the Sense of Reality* (Oxford University Press, 2008), 287, emphasis in original.

63. J. A. C. J. Bastiaansen et al., "Evidence for Mirror Systems in Emotions," *Philosophical Transactions of the Royal Society of London, B: Biological Sciences* 364, no. 1528 (2009): 2391–404.

64. Victoria Pitts-Taylor, *The Brain's Body: Neuroscience and Corporeal Politics* (Duke University Press, 2016), 91–93.

65. Jennifer E. Dayner et al., "Medical Treatment of Intersex: Parental Perspectives," *Journal of Urology* 172, no. 4 (2004): 1763. The authors surveyed the parents of twenty-one children.

66. Carolyn Pedwell, "Theorizing 'African' Female Genital Cutting and 'Western' Body Modifications: A Critique of the Continuum and Analogue Approaches," *Feminist Review* 86, no. 1 (2007): 64.

67. Merleau-Ponty, *The Visible and the Invisible*, 138.

68. Ailie J. Turton and Stuart R. Butler, "Referred Sensations Following Stroke," *Neurocase* 7, no. 5 (2001): 397–405.

69. V. S. Ramachandran and William Hirstein, "The Perception of Phantom Limbs," *Brain* 121, no. 9 (1998): 1603–30.

2. RUSHING TO TRAUMA

1. Chase, "What Is the Agenda of the Intersex Patient Advocacy Movement?," 240. The mission statement referring to trauma first appeared on ISNA's website in 2002 (https://www.isna.org). ISNA closed in 2008.

2. Daniela Truffer, "It's a Human Rights Issue!," *Narrative Inquiry in Bioethics* 5, no. 2 (2015): 113.

3. Garry Warne et al., "A Long-Term Outcome Study of Intersex Conditions," *Journal of Pediatric Endocrinology and Metabolism* 18, no. 6

(2005): 556; Katherine Rossiter and Shonna Diehl, "Gender Reassignment in Children: Ethical Conflicts in Surrogate Decision Making," *Pediatric Nursing* 24, no. 1 (1998): 59–60.

4. I am aware that some nonsurgical procedures, such as childhood vaginal dilation, can be traumatic, too; however, my focus in this chapter is primarily on surgery. For an early critique of childhood vaginal dilation as similar to sexual abuse, see Kessler, *Lessons from the Intersexed*, 63. Most clinicians no longer recommend performing such dilations in childhood, although that does not negate their impact on previous generations of patients.

5. Davis, *Contesting Intersex*, 28–43.

6. Feder, *Making Sense of Intersex*, 125.

7. Melinda Jones, "Intersex Genital Mutilation—a Western Version of FGM," *International Journal of Children's Rights* 25, no. 2 (2017): 396–411.

8. Alice Domurat Dreger, "Intersex Treatment as Standard Medical Practice, or, How Wrong I Was," *Medical Humanities Report* 24, no. 3 (2003): 1–4.

9. Arlene Istar Lev, "Intersexuality in the Family: An Unacknowledged Trauma," *Journal of Gay and Lesbian Psychotherapy* 10, no. 2 (2006): 39.

10. Moonhawk River Stone, "Approaching Critical Mass: An Exploration of the Role of Intersex Allies in Creative Positive Education, Advocacy, and Change," *Cardozo Journal of Law and Gender* 12, no. 1 (2005): 359.

11. For example, Katinka Schweizer et al., "Coping with Diverse Sex Development: Treatment Experiences and Psychosocial Support During Childhood and Adolescence and Adult Well-Being," *Journal of Pediatric Psychology* 42, no. 5 (2017): 513–14; Vickie Pasterski, Kiki Mastroyannopoulou, et al., "Predictors of Posttraumatic Stress in Parents of Children Diagnosed with a Disorder of Sex Development," *Archives of Sexual Behavior* 43, no. 2 (2014): 369–75. The latter authors reference the definition of post-traumatic stress syndrome in the American Psychiatric Association's *Diagnostic and Statistical Manual of Mental Disorders* (*DSM*), but their focus is on whether parents are traumatized by learning their child's intersex diagnosis rather than on trauma for the child. They suggest an intersex diagnosis could be traumatic

for parents because it is "a threat to the physical integrity of self or others," as the *DSM* puts it (quoted on 370). However, I argue that genital surgery is a much more salient threat to physical integrity.

12. Laura S. Brown, *Cultural Competence in Trauma Therapy: Beyond the Flashback* (American Psychological Association, 2008), 142–45.

13. As Katrina Roen puts it, "Psychological concerns are not in any way positioned so that they may bring the use of surgery into question." See Roen, "'But We Have to *Do Something*': Surgical 'Correction' of Atypical Genitalia," *Body & Society* 14, no. 1 (2008): 60.

14. M. Morgan Holmes, "Mind the Gaps: Intersex and (Re-Productive) Spaces in Disability Studies and Bioethics," *Bioethical Inquiry* 5, no. 2 (2008): 171.

15. Chase, "What Is the Agenda of the Intersex Patient Advocacy Movement?," 240. For an example of the traditionalist view, see Meyer-Bahlburg, "The Timing of Genital Surgery in Somatic Intersexuality," 13, 16, 17.

16. Esther Morris Leidolf, "The Missing Vagina Monologue . . . and Beyond," *Journal of Gay and Lesbian Psychotherapy* 10, no. 2 (2006): 89.

17. Pidgeon Pagonis, "The Son They Never Had," *Narrative Inquiry in Bioethics* 5, no. 2 (2015): 105, emphasis in original.

18. Iain Morland, "Intersex Treatment and the Promise of Trauma," in *Gender and the Science of Difference: Cultural Politics of Contemporary Science and Medicine*, ed. Jill A. Fisher (Rutgers University Press, 2011), 153–58. The present chapter takes a different direction from this earlier essay, which focused on sex-reassignment surgeries. In that earlier essay, I also positioned Tamara Alexander's work differently. Later in this chapter, I discuss Alexander's paper on intersex and trauma and set out my latest thinking on how it relates to the development of intersex criticism.

19. Interview with Arlene (no last name), quoted in Brown, *Cultural Competence in Trauma Therapy*, 145.

20. William Reiner, "To Be Male or Female—That Is the Question," *Archives of Pediatrics and Adolescent Medicine* 151, no. 3 (1997): 224–25.

21. Alice Domurat Dreger, "Shifting the Paradigm of Intersex Treatment," Intersex Society of North America, 2003, https://isna.org /compare.

22. Viloria, *Born Both*, 111–13.

23. Preves, *Intersex and Identity*, 93, 140.

24. Dreger and Herndon, "Progress and Politics in the Intersex Rights Movement," 217.

25. Jennifer M. Crawford et al., "Results from a Pediatric Surgical Centre Justify Early Intervention in Disorders of Sex Development," *Journal of Pediatric Surgery* 44, no. 2 (2009): 416.

26. Chase, "What Is the Agenda of the Intersex Patient Advocacy Movement?," 242. As David Rubin has noted, ISNA's claim "presumes that stigma and trauma are clearly separable from, and have no causal or correlative relation to, gender as a multidirectional structure of power." See Rubin, *Intersex Matters*, 91.

27. Graham Ingham, "Mental Work in a Trauma Patient," in *Understanding Trauma: A Psychoanalytical Approach*, ed. Caroline Garland (Duckworth, 1998), 98.

28. See Ralph Harrington, "On the Tracks of Trauma: Railway Spine Reconsidered," *Journal of the Society for the Social History of Medicine* 16, no. 2 (2003): 209–23.

29. Kai T. Erikson, *Everything in Its Path: Destruction of Community in the Buffalo Creek Flood* (Simon and Schuster, 1976), 153.

30. Judith Butler, *Undoing Gender* (Routledge, 2004), 156.

31. For example, William Byne, "Developmental Endocrine Influences on Gender Identity: Implications for Management of Disorders of Sex Development," *Mount Sinai Journal of Medicine* 73, no. 7 (2006): 951, 955–56.

32. For example, S. Faisal Ahmed, Carlo Acerini, et al., "Re: Parental Choice on Normalising Cosmetic Genital Surgery" (letter), *British Medical Journal*, October 8, 2015, https://www.bmj.com/content/351/bmj.h5124/rr-2.

33. Peter Hegarty et al., "Drawing the Line Between Essential and Nonessential Interventions on Intersex Characteristics with European Health Care Professionals," *Review of General Psychology* 25, no. 1 (2021): 101–14.

34. Jakub Mieszczak et al., "Assignment of the Sex of Rearing in the Neonate with a Disorder of Sex Development," *Current Opinion in Pediatrics* 21, no. 4 (2009): 544.

35. For a discussion of subjectivity along a different trajectory from that of the present chapter, see Morland, "Intersex Surgery Between the Gaze and the Subject."

36. Walid A. Farhat, "Early Intervention of CAH Surgical Management," *Journal of Pediatric and Adolescent Gynecology* 18, no. 1 (2005): 66; Rossiter and Diehl, "Gender Reassignment in Children," 61; Froukje M. E. Slijper et al., "Long-Term Psychological Evaluation of Intersex Children," *Archives of Sexual Behavior* 27, no. 2 (1998): 127.

37. Pierre D. E. Mouriquand, Daniela Brindusa Gorduza, et al., "Surgery in Disorders of Sex Development (DSD) with a Gender Issue: If (Why), When, and How?," *Journal of Pediatric Urology* 12, no. 3 (2016): 140.

38. On surgery being in the interests of the child as a gendered subject, see Joint LWPES/ESPE CAH Working Group, "Consensus Statement on 21-Hydroxylase Deficiency from the Lawson Wilkins Pediatric Endocrine Society and the European Society for Paediatric Endocrinology," *Journal of Clinical Endocrinology and Metabolism* 87, no. 9 (2002): 4050; and Walter L. Miller et al., "Authors' Response: Regarding the Consensus Statement on 21-Hydroxylase Deficiency from the Lawson Wilkins Pediatric Endocrine Society and the European Society for Paediatric Endocrinology," *Journal of Clinical Endocrinology and Metabolism* 88, no. 7 (2003): 3456. On surgery fulfilling a desire for gender regardless of the child's interests, see Claire Nihoul-Fékété, "Does Surgical Genitoplasty Affect Gender Identity in the Intersex Infant?," *Hormone Research* 64, supp. 2 (2005): 24.

39. For example, Rossiter and Diehl, "Gender Reassignment in Children," 60–61.

40. Cheryl Chase, "Hermaphrodites with Attitude: Mapping the Emergence of Intersex Political Activism," *GLQ* 4, no. 2 (1998): 189.

41. On this point, my account differs from Katrina Roen's analysis. Roen contrasts traditional medical depictions of "the young child as a malleable not-yet-subject" against reformist depictions of "the infant and the young child as embodied subjects." My focus in this chapter is on how both these ideas are incorporated in the practice of early genital surgery despite their incompatibility. See Roen, "Clinical Intervention

and Embodied Subjectivity: Atypically Sexed Children and Their Parents," in *Critical Intersex*, ed. Holmes, 32.

42. Tatiana Prade Hemesath et al., "Controversies on Timing of Sex Assignment and Surgery in Individuals with Disorders of Sex Development: A Perspective," *Frontiers in Pediatrics* 6 (2019): art. 419, https://doi.org/10.3389/fped.2018.00419, 3–4.

43. John Money et al., "Hermaphroditism: Recommendations Concerning Assignment of Sex, Change of Sex, and Psychologic Management," *Bulletin of the Johns Hopkins Hospital* 97, no. 4 (1955): 290.

44. Mendonca et al., "46,XY Disorders of Sex Development (DSD)," 183–84.

45. Slijper et al., "Long-Term Psychological Evaluation of Intersex Children," 132.

46. Brown, *Cultural Competence in Trauma Therapy*, 117–19.

47. Rossiter and Diehl, "Gender Reassignment in Children," 60. Endocrine Society guidelines suggest that "psychological trauma" would be caused by "genital surgery during childhood and adolescence," which can be avoided by doing surgery in infancy. See Speiser et al., "Congenital Adrenal Hyperplasia due to Steroid 21-Hydroxylase Deficiency," 4066.

48. Roberta Culbertson, "Embodied Memory, Transcendence, and Telling: Recounting Trauma, Re-Establishing the Self," *New Literary History* 26, no. 1 (1995): 171.

49. Candace Vogler, "Much of Madness and More of Sin: Compassion, for Ligeia," in *Compassion: The Culture and Politics of an Emotion*, ed. Lauren Berlant (Routledge: 2004), 41.

50. Marylene Cloitre et al., *Treating Survivors of Childhood Abuse: Psychotherapy for the Interrupted Life* (Guilford, 2006), 2.

51. Tamara Alexander, "The Medical Management of Intersexed Children: An Analogue for Childhood Sexual Abuse," Intersex Society of North America, 1997, https://isna.org/articles/analog, introduction and "Misinformation."

52. Alexander, "Medical Management of Intersexed Children," in the section titled "Dissociation and Body Estrangement."

53. Patricia K. Donahoe et al., "Clinical Management of Intersex Abnormalities," *Current Problems in Surgery* 28, no. 8 (1991): 553.

54. Alexander, "Medical Management of Intersexed Children," introduction.
55. Roger Luckhurst, "Traumaculture," *New Formations*, no. 50 (2003): 28.
56. Culbertson, "Embodied Memory," 175.
57. Hal Foster, "Death in America," *October*, no. 75 (1996): 37.
58. Within trauma studies, another way to think about the paradoxical status of the traumatized subject is in terms of mimesis and antimimesis. Understood as a problem of mimesis, trauma causes the subject to involuntarily imitate the traumatic scene or aggressor; understood as a problem of antimimesis, trauma causes the subject to detach from events that overwhelm it. As Ruth Leys has shown, the mimetic and antimimetic conceptions have existed in tension throughout the cultural history of trauma, shaping how trauma is treated as well as the perceived veracity of first-person accounts of traumatization. See Leys, *Trauma: A Genealogy* (University of Chicago Press, 2000), 8–10, 40.
59. Gil Eyal, "Identity and Trauma: Two Forms of the Will to Memory," *History and Memory* 16, no. 1 (2004): 11.
60. As the APA handbook on trauma therapy notes, "Varieties of childhood posttraumatic coping mechanisms, which frequently mask the damages done until later in life, have been mistaken for an absence of impact," although the handbook unfortunately does not apply this insight to the case of intersex treatment. Brown, *Cultural Competence in Trauma Therapy*, 117.
61. Holmes, *Intersex*, 166 n. 21.
62. Holmes, *Intersex*, 166 n. 21.
63. Farhat, "Early Intervention of CAH Surgical Management," 67.
64. Nihoul-Fékété, "How to Deal with Congenital Disorders of Sex Development in 2008 (DSD)," 367. Nihoul-Fékété also discusses the use of one-step surgeries for both feminization and masculinization (365).
65. K. P. Wolffenbuttel and Naomi S. Crouch, "Timing of Feminising Surgery in Disorders of Sex Development," in *Understanding Differences and Disorders of Sex Development (DSD)*, ed. Olaf Hiort and S. Faisal Ahmed (Karger, 2014), 219.
66. One of the leading proponents of dexamethasone for treating intersex, Maria New, is based at Mount Sinai, New York, where Holmes

gave the paper in the 1990s. For both sides of the debate about dexamethasone, see Maria New, "Description and Defense of Prenatal Diagnosis and Treatment with Low-Dose Dexamethasone for Congenital Adrenal Hyperplasia," *American Journal of Bioethics* 10, no. 9 (2010): 48–51; and Alice Domurat Dreger, Ellen K. Feder, et al., "Prenatal Dexamethasone for Congenital Adrenal Hyperplasia: An Ethics Canary in the Modern Medical Mine," *Bioethical Inquiry* 9, no. 3 (2012): 277–94.

3. HAUNTED ATTACHMENTS

1. Herman E. Stark, "Authenticity and Intersexuality," in *Ethics and Intersex*, ed. Sytsma, 274–77; Hazel Glenn Beh and Milton Diamond, "David Reimer's Legacy: Limiting Parental Discretion," *Cardozo Journal of Law and Gender* 12, no. 1 (2005): 5.
2. This complaint is indicative of a wider trend in Western modernity toward treating "anything damaging to the self or restricting it from being fully acknowledged, developed and expressed" as "a wrong that has to be fought," as Geertje Mak describes it. See Mak, *Doubting Sex*, 232.
3. Hilde Lindemann, "The Power of Parents and the Agency of Children," in *Surgically Shaping Children: Technology, Ethics, and the Pursuit of Normality*, ed. Erik Parens (Johns Hopkins University Press, 2006), 177–78.
4. John Bowlby, *The Making and Breaking of Affectional Bonds* (1979; Routledge, 2005), 139–40.
5. Govind B. Chavhan et al., "Imaging of Ambiguous Genitalia: Classification and Diagnostic Approach," *RadioGraphics* 28, no. 7 (2008): 1892; Cheryl Chase, "Rethinking Treatment for Ambiguous Genitalia," *Pediatric Nursing* 25, no. 4 (1999): 454.
6. I. A. Hughes et al., "Consensus Statement on Management of Intersex Disorders," *Archives of Disease in Childhood* 91, no. 7 (2006): 557.
7. Futoshi Matsui et al., "Long-Term Outcome of Ovotesticular Disorder of Sex Development: A Single Center Experience," *International Journal of Urology* 18, no. 3 (2011): 234; Caroline Sanders et al., "Searching for Harmony: Parents' Narratives About Their Child's Genital

Ambiguity and Reconstructive Genital Surgeries in Childhood," *Journal of Advanced Nursing* 67, no. 10 (2011): 2227.

8. Tamar-Mattis, "Exceptions to the Rule," 89–90, 101–2.

9. Ellen K. Feder, "Doctor's Orders: Parents and Intersexed Children," in *The Subject of Care: Feminist Perspectives on Dependency*, ed. Eva Feder Kittay and Ellen K. Feder (Rowman and Littlefield, 2002), 304.

10. Quoted in Sanders et al., "Parents' Narratives About Their Experiences of Their Child's Reconstructive Genital Surgeries," 3191.

11. Bowlby, *Making and Breaking of Affectional Bonds*, 84, 139, 126, 140.

12. As Lih-Mei Liao puts it poignantly, "The idea that normalizing surgery can ameliorate shame . . . comes with the message that the child, unaltered, is unlovable." See Liao, "Stonewalling Emotion," *Narrative Inquiry in Bioethics* 5, no. 2 (2015): 145.

13. The key theorists of these attachment styles are Mary Ainsworth and, of the disorganized style in particular, Mary Main. The ambivalent style is also known as the resistant style. For an overview, see David J. Wallin, *Attachment in Psychotherapy* (Guilford, 2007), 33.

14. For this reason, I avoid the custom of calling these styles "insecure" because it can imply that they are insubstantial or temporary.

15. Karen Zilberstein, "Neurocognitive Considerations in the Treatment of Attachment and Complex Trauma in Children," *Clinical Child Psychology and Psychiatry* 19, no. 3 (2014): 338.

16. Quoted in Halley P. Crissman et al., "Children with Disorders of Sex Development: A Qualitative Study of Early Parental Experiences," *International Journal of Pediatric Endocrinology* 2011: art. 10, https://doi.org/10.1186/1687-9856-2011-10, 5.

17. Quoted in Crissman et al., "Children with Disorders of Sex Development," 5.

18. For example, Karkazis, *Fixing Sex*, 212.

19. Margaret Simmonds, "Patients and Parents in Decision Making and Management," in *Paediatric and Adolescent Gynaecology: A Multidisciplinary Approach*, ed. Adam H. Balen et al. (Cambridge University Press, 2004), 216.

20. For an example of parents who chose not to have their child undergo normalizing surgery, see Lohman and Lohman, *Raising Rosie*.

21. Lev, "Intersexuality in the Family," 39.

22. Simmonds, "Patients and Parents in Decision Making and Management," 215–16.

23. Samantha Murray, "Within or Beyond the Binary/Boundary? Intersex Infants and Parental Decisions," *Australian Feminist Studies* 24, no. 60 (2009): 269.

24. Parents quoted in Crissman et al., "Children with Disorders of Sex Development," 5. Some researchers interpret parental reliance on decisions by medical staff as a "coping mechanism" for stress. See A. Duguid et al., "The Psychological Impact of Genital Anomalies on the Parents of Affected Children," *Acta Paediatrica* 96, no. 3 (2007): 350.

25. Jürgensen et al., "'Any Decision Is Better Than None,'" 363, 365.

26. Quoted in Crissman et al., "Children with Disorders of Sex Development," 4–5. Likewise, recent interviews with sixteen parents who chose clitoral surgery for their children found "no evidence of critical discussions with professionals or peers prior to or since their child's surgery." See Julie Alderson et al., "Why Do Parents Recommend Clitoral Surgery? Parental Perception of the Necessity, Benefit, and Cost of Early Childhood Clitoral Surgery for Congenital Adrenal Hyperplasia (CAH)," *International Journal of Impotence Research* 35, no. 1 (2023): 59.

27. Feder, "Doctor's Orders," 314.

28. Parents are quoted in Jenny Kleeman, "'We Don't Know If Your Baby's a Boy or a Girl': Growing Up Intersex," *The Guardian*, July 2, 2016, https://www.theguardian.com/world/2016/jul/02/male-and-female-what-is-it-like-to-be-intersex.

29. Quotes from Sanders et al., "Searching for Harmony," 2225; and Beh and Diamond, "David Reimer's Legacy," 6.

30. Quoted in Kleeman, "'We Don't Know If Your Baby's a Boy or a Girl.'"

31. Quoted in Sanders et al., "Parents' Narratives," 3192. For a summary of research into the actual attitudes of "the group who are feared to be the stigmatizers of people with intersex variations: the general public," see Peter Hegarty and Annette Smith, "Public Understanding of Intersex: An Update on Recent Findings," *International Journal of Impotence Research* 35, no. 1 (2023): 73.

32. Quotes from Sanders et al., "Searching for Harmony," 2225; Beh and Diamond, "David Reimer's Legacy," 6; and Kleeman, "'We Don't Know If Your Baby's a Boy or a Girl.'"

33. Quotes from Beh and Diamond, "David Reimer's Legacy," 6.
34. Limor Meoded Danon and Niza Yanay, "Intersexuality: On Secret Bodies and Secrecy," *Studies in Gender and Sexuality* 17, no. 1 (2016): 63.
35. For example, in a study across ten American hospitals, the parents of twenty-five of twenty-six affected children chose genital surgery. See Rebecca E. H. Ellens et al., "Psychological Adjustment of Parents of Children Born with Atypical Genitalia 1 Year After Genitoplasty," *Journal of Urology* 198, no. 4 (2017): 914–20.
36. Quotes from Beh and Diamond, "David Reimer's Legacy," 6; and Sanders et al., "Parents' Narratives," 3192.
37. Jürgensen et al., "'Any Decision Is Better Than None,'" 364; Matsui et al., "Long-Term Outcome of Ovotesticular Disorder of Sex Development," 236.
38. Shankarnarayan Srinath, "Identificatory Processes in Trauma," in *Understanding Trauma*, ed. Garland, 142.
39. Maria Torok, "Story of Fear: The Symptoms of Phobia—the Return of the Repressed or the Return of the Phantom?" (1975), in Nicolas Abraham and Maria Torok, *The Shell and the Kernel: Renewals of Psychoanalysis*, ed. and trans. Nicholas T. Rand (University of Chicago Press, 1994), 183. By Torok's interpretation, the absent person was Sigmund Freud himself, whom the boy later met in the course of psychoanalytic treatment. Torok describes Freud's role in the bath time scene as that of a "phantom," a concept that I explore later in this chapter. For the original case, see Sigmund Freud, "Analyse der Phobie eines fünfjährigen Knaben," in *Gesammelte Werke*, vol. 7 (Imago, 1941), 255. The word *Schweinerei* is translated too literally as "piggish" in the English *Standard Edition* of Freud's works. Torok's translator renders it more aptly as "dirty," which aligns with the other word used by the mother in the conversation at bath time (*unanständig*, or "indecent").
40. Chavhan et al., "Imaging of Ambiguous Genitalia," 1892; Claudia Wiesemann et al., "Ethical Principles and Recommendations for the Medical Management of Differences of Sex Development (DSD)/ Intersex in Children and Adolescents," *European Journal of Pediatrics* 169, no. 6 (2010): 674.

41. Quoted in Meira Weiss, "Fence Sitters: Parents' Reactions to Sexual Ambiguities in Their Newborn Children," *Semiotica* 107, nos. 1–2 (1995): 39–40.

42. Although medical guidelines have shifted toward disclosure in place of the past's outright lies (such as describing testes as ovaries), make no mistake: parents do not choose normalizing surgery because they want to talk about intersex. They choose surgery to *avoid* talking about it. See P. T. Cohen-Kettenis, "Psychosocial and Psychosexual Aspects of Disorders of Sex Development," *Best Practice & Research Clinical Endocrinology & Metabolism* 24, no. 2 (2010): 328.

43. Esther Rashkin, *Unspeakable Secrets and the Psychoanalysis of Culture* (State University of New York Press, 2008), 106.

44. On repression, see Sigmund Freud, "Repression" (1915), in *On the History of the Psycho-Analytic Movement, Papers on Metapsychology, and Other Works*, vol. 14 of *The Standard Edition of the Complete Psychological Works of Sigmund Freud*, ed. and trans. James Strachey (Hogarth, 1957), 147.

45. Crawford et al., "Results from a Pediatric Surgical Centre," 414.

46. Crouch and Creighton, "Long-Term Functional Outcomes of Female Genital Reconstruction in Childhood," 404. Traditionalists also assert that childhood amnesia means that patients do not remember "traumatic hospital experiences." See Crawford et al., "Results from a Pediatric Surgical Centre," 414. I critique this idea in chapter 2.

47. Carole Peterson, "Children's Long-Term Memory for Autobiographical Events," *Developmental Review* 22, no. 3 (2002): 384.

48. Two examples of medical authors on intersex not engaging with the literature on childhood memory are Crawford et al., "Results from a Pediatric Surgical Centre," and Crouch and Creighton, "Long-Term Functional Outcomes of Female Genital Reconstruction in Childhood." Despite their different conclusions, both articles make generalized claims about childhood amnesia without citing relevant work in developmental psychology.

49. Peterson, "Children's Long-Term Memory," 372, 376.

50. Brendan C. Jones et al., "Early Hypospadias Surgery May Lead to a Better Long-Term Psychosexual Outcome," *Journal of Urology* 182, supp. 4 (2009): 1748.

51. Nicolas Abraham, "Seminar on Dual Unity and the Phantom" (1978), trans. Tom Goodwin, *Diacritics* 44, no. 4 (2016): 16.

52. Harold P. Blum, "Separation-Individuation Theory and Attachment Theory," *Journal of the American Psychoanalytic Association* 52, no. 2 (2004): 550–51, 540. My focus here is on Abraham and Torok, but the most prominent psychoanalytic theorist of dual unity and individuation is Margaret Mahler, as discussed by Blum.

53. Abraham, "Seminar on Dual Unity and the Phantom," 26.

54. Torok, "Story of Fear," 181.

55. Esther Rashkin, *Family Secrets and the Psychoanalysis of Narrative* (Princeton University Press, 1992), 17, 21.

56. Sigmund Freud, "The Unconscious" (1915), in Freud, *On the History of the Psycho-Analytic Movement*, 201, 202.

57. Abraham, "Seminar on Dual Unity and the Phantom," 26.

58. Rashkin, *Family Secrets*, 18.

59. Torok, "Story of Fear," 180.

60. Nicolas Abraham and Maria Torok, "'The Lost Object—Me': Notes on Endocryptic Identification" (1975), in Abraham and Torok, *The Shell and the Kernel*, 140 n. 1.

61. Quoted in Drew MacKenzie et al., "The Experiences of People with an Intersex Condition: A Journey from Silence to Voice," *Journal of Clinical Nursing* 18, no. 12 (2009): 1778.

62. Nicolas Abraham, "Notes on the Phantom: A Complement to Freud's Metapsychology" (1975), in Abraham and Torok, *The Shell and the Kernel*, 173.

63. Torok, "Story of Fear," 181. The phantom in this psychoanalytic sense depends on the existence of the unconscious, so it is different from Celeste Orr's conception of intersex in general as "an elusive queering, cripping ghost that tells us that our body-minds are not transparently or definitively sexed, dis/ordered, or gendered." See Orr, *Cripping Intersex*, 116.

64. Rashkin, *Unspeakable Secrets*, 94.

65. Robyn Fivush and Katherine Nelson, "Culture and Language in the Emergence of Autobiographical Memory," *Psychological Science* 15, no. 9 (2004): 574–75; Peterson, "Children's Long-Term Memory," 384, 393; Katherine Nelson, "The Psychological and Social

Origins of Autobiographical Memory," *Psychological Science* 4, no. 1 (1993): 10.

66. Quoted in Sanders et al., "Parents' Narratives," 3192.
67. Torok, "Story of Fear," 183.
68. Mary Main et al., "Security in Infancy, Childhood, and Adulthood: A Move to the Level of Representation," *Monographs of the Society for Research in Child Development* 50, nos. 1–2 (1985): 86; Peterson, "Children's Long-Term Memory," 393.
69. Rashkin, *Unspeakable Secrets*, 95.

4. WHAT CAN QUEER THEORY DO FOR INTERSEX?

1. Sarah E. Chinn, "Feeling Her Way: Audre Lorde and the Power of Touch," *GLQ* 9, nos. 1–2 (2003): 192, 182.
2. Cheryl Chase, "Re: Measurement of Pudendal Evoked Potentials During Feminizing Genitoplasty: Technique and Applications" (letter), *Journal of Urology* 156, no. 3 (1996): 1139, 1140.
3. Naomi S. Crouch et al., "Genital Sensation After Feminizing Genitoplasty for Congenital Adrenal Hyperplasia: A Pilot Study," *BJU International* 93, no. 1 (2004): 137.
4. Crouch et al., "Genital Sensation After Feminizing Genitoplasty," 138.
5. J. P. Gearhart et al., "In Reply: Re: Measurement of Pudendal Evoked Potentials During Feminizing Genitoplasty: Technique and Applications" (letter), *Journal of Urology* 156, no. 3 (1996): 1140.
6. Lee Edelman, "Queer Theory: Unstating Desire," *GLQ* 2, no. 4 (1995): 344.
7. On the feminist critique of sexual pleasure, see Wendy Hollway, "Theorizing Heterosexuality: A Response," *Feminism & Psychology* 3, no. 3 (1993): 412–17.
8. Patrick Califia (as Pat Califia), "A Secret Side of Lesbian Sexuality" (1979), in *Public Sex: The Culture of Radical Sex*, 2nd ed. (Cleis, 2000), 166.
9. Chase, "Affronting Reason," 210, emphasis in original.
10. For example, Betsy Driver, preface to special issue on intersex, *Cardozo Journal of Law and Gender* 12, no. 1 (2005): 3; Peter Hegarty and Cheryl

Chase, "Intersex Activism, Feminism, and Psychology" (2000), in *Queer Theory*, ed. Iain Morland and Annabelle Willox (Palgrave, 2005), 80; M. Morgan Holmes, "Queer Cut Bodies," in *Queer Frontiers: Millennial Geographies, Genders, and Generations*, ed. Joseph A. Boone et al. (University of Wisconsin Press, 2000), 98; Emi Koyama, *Intersex Critiques: Notes on Intersex, Disability, and Biomedical Ethics* (Confluere, 2003), 3, 7, 15; Malatino, *Queer Embodiment*, 141.

11. John P. Gearhart in M. M. Bailez et al., "Vaginal Reconstruction After Initial Construction of the External Genitalia in Girls with Salt-Wasting Adrenal Hyperplasia," *Journal of Urology* 148, no. 2 (1992): 684; Terry W. Hensle et al., "Sexual Function Following Bowel Vaginoplasty," *Journal of Urology* 175, no. 6 (2006): 2284. Bailez and coauthors also complain that one patient "needs an additional reconstructive operation but refuses additional therapy and reports homosexual activity only" (681).

12. Lee, Nordenström, et al., "Global Disorders of Sex Development Update Since 2006," 169. For a critique of research claims about intersex and "sex-typed interests," see Rebecca M. Jordan-Young, *Brain Storm: The Flaws in the Science of Sex Differences* (Harvard University Press, 2010), 203–13.

13. Stephen Whittle, "Gender Fucking or Fucking Gender?" (1996), in *Queer Theory*, ed. Morland and Willox, 126.

14. Douglas Crimp, "Melancholia and Moralism," in *Loss: The Politics of Mourning*, ed. David L. Eng and David Kazanjian (University of California Press, 2002), 199.

15. Patrick Califia (as Pat Califia), "Genderbending: Playing with Roles and Reversals" (1983), in Califia, *Public Sex*, 185. The most influential articulation of resignification as a feminist/queer practice is Judith Butler, *Gender Trouble: Feminism and the Subversion of Identity*, 2nd ed. (Routledge, 2006), 45.

16. Tony Snow, "Straight Sex Cannot Give You AIDS—Official," *Sun* (UK), November 17, 1989; Opendra Narayan quoted in Leo Bersani, "Is the Rectum a Grave?," in *AIDS: Cultural Analysis, Cultural Activism*, ed. Douglas Crimp (MIT Press, 1988), 197.

17. David M. Halperin, *Saint Foucault: Towards a Gay Hagiography* (Oxford University Press, 1995), 26. Halperin's account has some

limitations, demonstrated by the suggestion that "Foucault's focus on sexuality, and his refusal to subordinate the analysis of its instrumentality to the politics of gender, race, or class, made his work particularly useful for addressing the irreducibly *sexual* politics of the AIDS crisis" (27, emphasis in original). Although this engagement with Foucault's thought may be paradigmatically queer, it fails to consider how identity categories can intersect to create the appearance that they are irreducibly distinct—for example, when the intersection between the categories "white" and "gay" can produce a perspective from which sexuality appears (falsely) to be entirely unmarked by "race." See Damien W. Riggs, *Priscilla, (White) Queen of the Desert: Queer Rights/Race Privilege* (Peter Lang, 2006).

18. Halperin, *Saint Foucault*, 27, 28.

19. Michel Foucault, *The Will to Knowledge*, vol. 1 of *The History of Sexuality* (1976), trans. Robert Hurley (Penguin, 1978), 155, 157. I explore Foucault's account of power and knowledge further in chapter 5.

20. Lauren Berlant and Elizabeth Freeman, "Queer Nationality," in Lauren Berlant, *The Queen of America Goes to Washington City: Essays on Sex and Citizenship* (Duke University Press, 1997), 158.

21. Tim Dean, *Beyond Sexuality* (University of Chicago Press, 2000), 172.

22. Mark Blasius, *Gay and Lesbian Politics: Sexuality and the Emergence of a New Ethic* (Temple University Press, 1994), 110; Halperin, *Saint Foucault*, 28. On the "queerness" of Blasius's "new ethic," see *Gay and Lesbian Politics*, 125, 221.

23. Michel Foucault, "Sex, Power, and the Politics of Identity" (1984), interview by B. Gallagher and A. Wilson, in *Ethics: Subjectivity and Truth*, vol. 1 of *The Essential Works of Foucault, 1954–1984*, ed. Paul Rabinow, trans. Robert Hurley et al. (New Press, 1997), 164–65.

24. Amber Hollibaugh in Deirdre English et al., "Talking Sex: A Conversation on Sexuality and Feminism," *Feminist Review*, no. 11 (1982): 44.

25. Chase, "Affronting Reason," 207.

26. Sally R. Munt, "Shame/Pride Dichotomies in *Queer as Folk*," *Textual Practice* 14, no. 3 (2000): 533, 536.

27. Bersani, "Is the Rectum a Grave?," 197–98, 222.

28. Kathryn Bond Stockton, *Beautiful Bottom, Beautiful Shame: Where "Black" Meets "Queer"* (Duke University Press, 2006), 15.
29. Bersani, "Is the Rectum a Grave?," 222, 212.
30. Robert L. Caserio, "The Antisocial Thesis in Queer Theory," *PMLA* 121, no. 3 (2006): 819–21.
31. Leo Bersani, *Homos* (Harvard University Press, 1995), 93; see also 94.
32. Stockton, *Beautiful Bottom*, 15. The antisocial relationship between negativity and futurity has been explored most polemically by Lee Edelman in *No Future: Queer Theory and the Death Drive* (Duke University Press, 2004).
33. Michael Warner, *The Trouble with Normal: Sex, Politics, and the Ethics of Queer Life* (Harvard University Press, 1999), 35, 36, emphasis in original.
34. Bersani, *Homos*, 35.
35. Bersani, *Homos*, 80; Stockton, *Beautiful Bottom*, 15.
36. Heather Love, *Feeling Backward: Loss and the Politics of Queer History* (Harvard University Press, 2007), 40. However, Love does ultimately seem to recuperate as "bound up with pleasure" the emotions associated with an aversion to sex (161).
37. Love, *Feeling Backward*, 175 n. 22.
38. Jack Halberstam (as Judith Halberstam), "Lesbian Masculinity, or Even Stone Butches Get the Blues," *Women and Performance* 8, no. 2 (1996): 64, 68.
39. Halberstam, "Lesbian Masculinity," 63, 68, 69.
40. Feder, "Imperatives of Normality."
41. For further discussion of the inclusion of intersex under the LGBTQI+ umbrella, see Monro et al., *Intersex, Variations of Sex Characteristics, and DSD*, 46–48.
42. Ann Cvetkovich, *An Archive of Feelings: Trauma, Sexuality, and Lesbian Public Cultures* (Duke University Press, 2003), 67.
43. Ashley Montagu, *Touching: The Human Significance of the Skin* (Columbia University Press, 1971), 292.
44. Shildrick, "Unreformed Bodies," 329.
45. Chinn, "Feeling Her Way," 195; Margrit Shildrick, *Embodying the Monster: Encounters with the Vulnerable Self* (Sage, 2002), 119; Iris Marion Young, "The Scaling of Bodies and the Politics of Identity" (1990),

in *Space, Gender, Knowledge: Feminist Readings*, ed. Linda McDowell and Joanne P. Sharp (Arnold, 1997), 221.

46. Carolyn Dinshaw, "Chaucer's Queer Touches/A Queer Touches Chaucer," *Exemplaria* 7, no. 1 (1995): 75–92.

47. Warner, *The Trouble with Normal*, 36.

48. Patrick Califia (as Pat Califia), "Gay Men, Lesbians, and Sex: Doing It Together" (1983), in Califia, *Public Sex*, 194.

49. Elizabeth Freeman, "Time Binds, or, Erotohistoriography," *Social Text* 23, nos. 3–4 (2005): 66, emphasis in original.

50. Lauren Berlant, "'68 or The Revolution of Little Queers," in *Feminism Beside Itself*, ed. Diane Elam and Robyn Wiegman (Routledge, 1995), 301.

51. Lauren Berlant and Michael Warner, "Sex in Public" (1998), in Michael Warner, *Publics and Counterpublics* (Zone, 2002), 207–8.

52. Dinshaw, "Chaucer's Queer Touches," 92, 89, 79, 76, 77.

53. Dinshaw, "Chaucer's Queer Touches," 79.

54. Pearl Katz provides a seminal account of the stylized aspects of the operating room in "Ritual in the Operating Room," *Ethnology* 20, no. 4 (1981): 335–50.

55. Sara Ahmed, *The Cultural Politics of Emotion* (Edinburgh University Press, 2004), 27.

56. Esther Newton, *Mother Camp: Female Impersonators in America* (University of Chicago Press, 1979), 101.

57. Dreger, *Hermaphrodites*, 200.

58. Lih-Mei Liao, "Learning to Assist Women Born with Atypical Genitalia: Journey Through Ignorance, Taboo, and Dilemma," *Journal of Reproductive and Infant Psychology* 21, no. 3 (2003): 233. Such unease and avoidance may further diminish genital tactility by lowering arousability; see Kenneth J. Zucker et al., "Self-Reported Sexual Arousability in Women with Congenital Adrenal Hyperplasia," *Journal of Sex and Marital Therapy* 30, no. 5 (2004): 350–52.

59. Liao, *Variations in Sex Development*, 237.

60. Holmes, *Intersex*, 154.

61. For an example of medical rhetoric about "harsh teasing and ridicule, if not outright abuse" in the locker room, see Daaboul and Frader, "Ethics and the Management of the Patient with Intersex," 1581.

62. Elizabeth Freeman, "Packing History, Count(er)ing Generations," *New Literary History* 31, no. 4 (2000): 728, 729.

63. Ahmed, *Cultural Politics*, 25.

64. Gayle Salamon, "Boys of the Lex: Transgenderism and Rhetorics of Materiality," *GLQ* 12, no. 4 (2006): 583.

65. Jack Halberstam (as Judith Halberstam), *In a Queer Time and Place: Transgender Bodies, Subcultural Lives* (New York University Press, 2005), 2.

66. Jack Halberstam (as Judith Halberstam) in Carolyn Dinshaw et al., "Theorizing Queer Temporalities: A Roundtable Discussion," *GLQ* 13, nos. 2–3 (2007): 190.

67. Dinshaw, "Chaucer's Queer Touches," 79; Carolyn Dinshaw, *Getting Medieval: Sexualities and Communities, Pre- and Postmodern* (Duke University Press, 1999), 21.

68. My focus here on the postsurgical body is therefore different from that of David Andrew Griffiths, whose response to the earlier published version of this chapter addresses the possibility of "queer potential for pleasure" in a future when genital surgery is postponed "endlessly." See Griffiths, "Queering the Moment of Hypospadias 'Repair,'" *GLQ* 27, no. 4 (2021): 516, 517; and Iain Morland, "What Can Queer Theory Do for Intersex?," *GLQ: A Journal of Lesbian and Gay Studies* 15, no. 2 (2009): 285–312.

69. Amber Hollibaugh, "My Dangerous Desires: Falling in Love with Stone Butches, Passing Women, and Girls (Who Are Guys) Who Catch My Eye" (2000), in *Queer Cultures*, ed. Deborah Carlin and Jennifer DiGrazia (Pearson Prentice Hall, 2004), 383.

70. Donald Morton, "Birth of the Cyberqueer," *PMLA* 110, no. 3 (1995): 375, 372.

71. Salamon, "Boys of the Lex," 583.

72. Morton, "Birth of the Cyberqueer," 369. In chapter 6, I demonstrate a different kind of historical materialist analysis of intersex medicine.

73. Quoted in John Colapinto, *As Nature Made Him: The Boy Who Was Raised as a Girl* (Quartet, 2000), 148. For a full account of the Reimer case in relation to intersex treatment, see Morland, "Gender, Genitals, and the Meaning of Being Human."

74. Morton, "Birth of the Cyberqueer," 371.

75. Edelman, "Queer Theory," 345.

5. IN SEARCH OF MEDICAL POWER

1. Jemima Repo, *The Biopolitics of Gender* (Oxford University Press, 2016), 24–48.

2. Emily Grabham, "Citizen Bodies, Intersex Citizenship," *Sexualities* 10, no. 1 (2007): 40.

3. Milton Diamond and Jameson Garland, "Evidence Regarding Cosmetic and Medically Unnecessary Surgery on Infants," *Journal of Pediatric Urology* 10, no. 1 (2014): 2–7.

4. Ute Lampalzer et al., "Dealing with Uncertainty and Lack of Knowledge in Diverse Sex Development: Controversies on Early Surgery and Questions of Consent," *Sexual Medicine* 8, no. 3 (2020): 479.

5. Pierre D. E. Mouriquand, Anthony C. Caldamone, et al., "The ESPU/SPU Standpoint on the Surgical Management of Disorders of Sex Development (DSD)," *Journal of Pediatric Urology* 10, no. 1 (2014): 10.

6. Dayner et al., "Medical Treatment of Intersex," 1762; Sarah M. Creighton et al., "Objective Cosmetic and Anatomical Outcomes at Adolescence of Feminising Surgery for Ambiguous Genitalia Done in Childhood," *Lancet* 358, no. 9276 (2001): 124.

7. Richard J. Auchus et al., "Guidelines for the Development of Comprehensive Care Centers for Congenital Adrenal Hyperplasia: Guidance from the CARES Foundation Initiative," *International Journal of Pediatric Endocrinology* 2010: art. 275213, https://doi.org/10.1155/2010/275213, 11.

8. Sean Saifa Wall, "Standing at the Intersections: Navigating Life as a Black Intersex Man," *Narrative Inquiry in Bioethics* 5, no. 2 (2015): 117.

9. Fausto-Sterling, "The Five Sexes," 24.

10. Nancy Ehrenreich, with Mark Barr, "Intersex Surgery, Female Genital Cutting, and the Selective Condemnation of 'Cultural Practices,'" *Harvard Civil Rights–Civil Liberties Law Review* 40, no. 1 (2005): 114. On this point, some activists and critics have deployed the discipline frame to reframe medical interventions as human rights abuses. See Daniela Crocetti, Elia A. G. Arfini, et al., "'You're Basically

Calling Doctors Torturers': Stakeholder Framing Issues Around Naming Intersex Rights Claims as Human Rights Abuses," *Sociology of Health & Illness* 42, no. 4 (2020): 949–51.

11. Sungchan Park et al., "Long-Term Follow-up After Feminizing Genital Reconstruction in Patients with Ambiguous Genitalia and High Vaginal Confluence," *Journal of Korean Medical Science* 26, no. 3 (2011): 400.

12. Malatino, *Queer Embodiment*, 163.

13. Mostafa M. Ali et al., "Results of Two-Stage Transverse Preputial Island Flap Urethroplasty for Proximal Hypospadias with Chordee That Mandate Division of the Urethral Plate," *Central European Journal of Urology* 74, no. 1 (2021): 90.

14. Anne Fausto-Sterling, *Sexing the Body: Gender Politics and the Construction of Sexuality* (Basic, 2000), 40.

15. Chase, "Affronting Reason," 209.

16. Theocharis Papageorgiou et al., "Clitoroplasty with Preservation of Neurovascular Pedicles," *Obstetrics and Gynecology* 96, no. 5 (2000): 822.

17. Sherri A. Groveman, "The Hanukkah Bush: Ethical Implications in the Clinical Management of Intersex," in *Intersex in the Age of Ethics*, ed. Dreger, 27.

18. Elizabeth Reilly, "Radical Tweak—Relocating the Power to Assign Sex," *Cardozo Journal of Law and Gender* 12, no. 1 (2005): 303–4.

19. Myra J. Hird and Jenz Germon, "The Intersexual Body and the Medical Regulation of Gender," in *Constructing Gendered Bodies*, ed. Kathryn Backett-Milburn and Linda McKie (Palgrave, 2001), 174.

20. Park et al., "Long-Term Follow-up After Feminizing Genital Reconstruction," 402.

21. Katie Goss, "Intersex's New Materialism: More-Than-Binary Bio-Logics in Lucia Puenzo's *XXY*," *Transgender Studies Quarterly* 9, no. 2 (2022): 238.

22. Jules Gill-Peterson (as Julian Gill-Peterson) calls this corporeal agency "the partially autonomous nonhuman agency expressed in embodied plasticity." See Gill-Peterson, *Histories of the Transgender Child*, 113.

23. Holmes, "Queer Cut Bodies," in *Queer Frontiers*, ed. Boone et al., 103, emphasis in original.

24. Ali et al., "Results of Two-Stage Transverse Preputial Island Flap Urethroplasty," 93.

25. Holmes, "Queer Cut Bodies," in *Queer Frontiers*, ed. Boone et al., 91.

26. David, "I Am Not Alone!," *Hermaphrodites with Attitudes*, Winter 1994, https://isna.org/files/hwa/winter1995.pdf, 5.

27. Papageorgiou et al., "Clitoroplasty," 821.

28. Thomas E. Wartenberg, *The Forms of Power: From Domination to Transformation* (Temple University Press, 1990), 17–26.

29. There is also a debate in social theory about whether one can possess power merely by having the *capacity* to do something, irrespective of whether one does it, but my discussion in this chapter focuses on the power exercised through medical practices because that is the key point of contention with regard to intersex management. See Wartenberg, *Forms of Power*, 22–23.

30. Thelma Wang, "Trans as Brain Intersex: The Trans–Intersex Nexus in Neurobiological Research," *Transgender Studies Quarterly* 9, no. 2 (2022): 177.

31. Meoded Danon and Yanay, "Intersexuality," 57.

32. Michel Foucault, "Powers and Strategies" (1977), interview by Jean Borreil et al., in *Power/Knowledge: Selected Interviews and Other Writings, 1972–1977*, ed. and trans. Colin Gordon (Pantheon, 1980), 141.

33. Judith Butler, *Bodies That Matter: On the Discursive Limits of "Sex"* (Routledge, 1993), 9.

34. Zygmunt Bauman, *Liquid Modernity* (Polity, 2000), 6, 145, 29, 149, 14.

35. Tiger Devore (as Howard Devore), "Growing Up in the Surgical Maelstrom," in *Intersex in the Age of Ethics*, ed. Dreger, 80.

36. Meoded Danon and Yanay, "Intersexuality," 58.

37. Georgiann Davis and Erin L. Murphy have theorized this operation in terms of the philosopher Giorgio Agamben's concept of the state of exception, whereby the body becomes the site from which its own intersex traits are excluded. See Davis and Murphy, "Intersex Bodies as States of Exception: An Empirical Explanation for Unnecessary Surgical Modification," *Feminist Formations* 25, no. 2 (2013): 134.

38. Meoded Danon and Yanay, "Intersexuality," 58, 70.

39. John Money's highly influential publications in this field recommended that in the event of surgical sex reassignment, parents should enlist a local "public figure" such as a pastor, doctor, or lawyer to

explain to the community that their baby required medical intervention, before the parents show their baby's modified genitalia to others. See Money, *Sex Errors of the Body: Dilemmas, Education, Counseling* (Johns Hopkins University Press, 1968), 62.

40. Jo Bird, "Outside the Law: Intersex, Medicine, and the Discourse of Rights," *Cardozo Journal of Law and Gender* 12, no. 1 (2005): 79.

41. Michel Foucault, "Body/Power" (1975), interview by editorial collective of *Quel Corps?*, in Foucault, *Power/Knowledge*, 59.

42. One intersex woman recounted that when she obtained her medical records at age nineteen to understand why she had an abdominal scar, "it undermined me even more than I could have imagined. The file said 'hermaphrodite,' 'pseudo-hermaphrodite,' 'true hermaphrodite.' And then it had a boy's name that had been given to me crossed out and my girl's name written over it. And I thought: everyone else in my family knows this?" Quoted in Human Rights Watch, *"I Want to Be Like Nature Made Me,"* 34.

43. Luckhurst, "Traumaculture," 33–34; Nigel Thrift, *Spatial Formations* (Sage, 1996), 264–84. During this period, the rise of urban hospitals and development of anesthetic meant that encounters between doctors and individuals with intersex anatomies became more impersonal, too. Hospital-based consultations meant that medical knowledge was disconnected from the lives that patients lived in their communities, and examinations under anesthetic generated medical knowledge that was radically different from what patients knew about their own bodies. See Mak, *Doubting Sex*, 42, 99, 136.

44. Bauman, *Liquid Modernity*, 148–49, 163.

45. Iain Morland, "Cybernetic Sexology," in Downing et al., *Fuckology*, 101–32. My argument in the present chapter is specifically about the ways of treating intersex that originated in the middle of the twentieth century. The argument I am making here does not negate the medicalization of intersex in other periods, including earlier efforts at genital surgery, such as those described by Leah DeVun in *The Shape of Sex: Nonbinary Gender from Genesis to the Renaissance* (Columbia University Press, 2021), 134–62.

46. Mark Seltzer, *Serial Killers: Death and Life in America's Wound Culture* (Routledge, 1998), 1, 254, 22.

47. Michel Foucault, "Prison Talk" (1975), interview by Jean-Jacques Brochier, in Foucault, *Power/Knowledge*, 52.

48. Peter A. Lee, Amy B. Wisniewski, et al., "Advances in Diagnosis and Care of Persons with DSD Over the Last Decade," *International Journal of Pediatric Endocrinology* 2014: art. 19, https://doi.org/10.1186/1687 -9856-2014-19, 5, 4.

49. Cools et al., "Caring for Individuals with a Difference of Sex Development (DSD)," 421.

50. Meoded Danon, "Temporal Sociomedical Approaches to Intersex* Bodies," 15. As Emily Grabham has observed, the concept of following up on complications from previous intersex surgeries "enables what would otherwise be classed as 'new' procedures and provides a justifying context for the associated risks of those procedures." See Grabham, "Bodily Integrity and the Surgical Management of Intersex," 13.

51. Bauman, *Liquid Modernity*, 11.

52. Stefan Timmermans et al., "Does Patient-Centered Care Change Genital Surgery Decisions? The Strategic Use of Clinical Uncertainty in Disorders of Sex Development Clinics," *Journal of Health and Social Behavior* 59, no. 4 (2018): 532.

53. S. Faisal Ahmed, Melissa Gardner, et al., "Management of Children with Disorders of Sex Development: New Care Standards Explained," *Psychology and Sexuality* 5, no. 1 (2014): 5.

54. Anonymous geneticist quoted in Lih-Mei Liao and Katrina Roen, "The Role of Psychologists in Multi-Disciplinary Teams for Intersex/ Diverse Sex Development: Interviews with British and Swedish Clinical Specialists," *Psychology and Sexuality* 12, no. 3 (2021): 206.

55. Quoted in Monro et al., *Intersex, Variations of Sex Characteristics, and DSD*, 29.

56. Jorge Daaboul in Martin T. Stein et al., "A Newborn Infant with a Disorder of Sexual Differentiation," *Pediatrics* 114, no. 5 (2004): 1476–77; Liao and Roen, "Role of Psychologists in Multi-Disciplinary Teams," 207.

57. Quoted in Monro et al., *Intersex, Variations of Sex Characteristics, and DSD*, 29.

58. Hüseyin Özbey and Seref Etker, "Disorders of Sexual Development in a Cultural Context," *Arab Journal of Urology* 11, no. 1 (2013): 34.

59. Mouriquand, Caldamone, et al., "ESPU/SPU Standpoint," 10.

60. Asia Friedman, *Blind to Sameness: Sexpectations and the Social Construction of Male and Female Bodies* (University of Chicago Press, 2013), 2.

61. Elizabeth Wingrove, "Interpellating Sex," *Signs* 24, no. 4 (1999): 879.

62. Lee, Nordenström, et al., "Global Disorders of Sex Development Update Since 2006," 177.

63. Bauman, *Liquid Modernity*, 7–8.

64. Lauren Berlant, "Compassion (and Withholding)," in *Compassion*, ed. Berlant, 6. The late-modern "liberal society that sanctions individuality as sovereign" (5) discussed by Berlant is the latest manifestation of "the prevalent tendency in bourgeois morality to lay exclusive value upon conviction" that Max Horkheimer identified earlier in the twentieth century. See Horkheimer, "Materialism and Morality" (1933), in *Between Philosophy and Social Science: Selected Early Writings*, trans. G. Frederick Hunter et al. (MIT Press, 1993), 24.

65. Cary Gabriel Costello, "Beyond Binary Sex and Gender Ideology," in *The Oxford Handbook of the Sociology of the Body and Embodiment*, ed. Natalie Boero and Katherine Mason (Oxford University Press, 2020), 204.

66. Louis Althusser, "Ideology and Ideological State Apparatuses (Notes Towards an Investigation)" (1970), in *Lenin and Philosophy, and Other Essays*, trans. Ben Brewster (NLB, 1971), 157. Althusser adds that subjects "work by themselves" (169).

67. Wingrove, "Interpellating Sex," 875.

68. Althusser, "Ideology and Ideological State Apparatuses," 151.

69. This effect is what Althusser refers to as an "imaginary relation to real relations." See Althusser, "Ideology and Ideological State Apparatuses," 156.

70. The nomenclature *preimplantation genetic testing* encompasses two earlier terms, *preimplantation genetic diagnosis* (PGD) and *preimplantation genetic screening* (PGS). See Firuza Rajesh Parikh et al., "Preimplantation Genetic Testing: Its Evolution, Where Are We Today?," *Journal of Human Reproductive Sciences* 11, no. 4 (2018): 309.

71. This is typically in the scenario where parents are aware of heritable conditions that can be detected by testing; however, in some countries it is also permissible for parents to select the sex of the embryos that

are implanted. See Miriam Bentwich, "On the Inseparability of Gender Eugenics, Ethics, and Public Policy: An Israeli Perspective," *American Journal of Bioethics* 13, no. 10 (2013): 44.

72. Robert Sparrow, "Gender Eugenics? The Ethics of PGD for Intersex Conditions," *American Journal of Bioethics* 13, no. 10 (2013): 31. Celeste Orr provides an extended critique of Sparrow's wider argument in *Cripping Intersex*, 219–31, 240–54.

73. This is similar to how some clinicians present prenatal steroidal treatments as a means to avoid feminizing surgeries. See Dreger, Feder, et al., "Prenatal Dexmethasone for Congenital Adrenal Hyperplasia," 281.

74. Sparrow, "Gender Eugenics?," 31.

75. Sparrow, "Gender Eugenics?," 36; Georgiann Davis, "The Social Costs of Preempting Intersex Traits," *American Journal of Bioethics* 13, no. 10 (2013): 52.

76. Laurence B. McCullough, "Critically Appraising Prenatal Genetic Diagnosis to Prevent Disorders of Sexual Development: An Opportunity Missed," *American Journal of Bioethics* 13, no. 10 (2013): 2.

77. As Nancy Fraser has noted, to cast matters as private as opposed to public is "to shield them from broadly based debate and contestation." See Fraser, "Rethinking the Public Sphere: A Contribution to the Critique of Actually Existing Democracy," in *Habermas and the Public Sphere*, ed. Craig Calhoun (MIT Press, 1992), 132.

6. WAS INTERSEX REAL?

1. Iain Morland, "Is Intersexuality Real?," *Textual Practice* 15, no. 3 (2001): 527–47.

2. Dreger, *Hermaphrodites*, 150–57; Morland, "Is Intersexuality Real?" On the longer history of representations of intersex as inauthentic, see DeVun, *The Shape of Sex*, 109, 119.

3. For example, Arnold G. Coran and Theodore Z. Polley Jr., "Surgical Management of Ambiguous Genitalia in the Infant and Child," *Journal of Pediatric Surgery* 26, no. 7 (1991): 818.

4. Swarr, *Envisioning African Intersex*, 39.

5. See Preves, *Intersex and Identity*, 89–98.

6. Colette St-Hilaire, "Crisis and Mutation of the Apparatus of Sexuality: The Bursting of the Category of Sex" (1999), trans. Jean Antonin Billard and Erin Mouré, *West Coast Line*, no. 35 (2001): 140.

7. Kessler, *Lessons from the Intersexed*, 128, 105.

8. Alice Domurat Dreger, Cheryl Chase, et al., "Changing the Nomenclature/Taxonomy for Intersex: A Scientific and Clinical Rationale," *Journal of Pediatric Endocrinology and Metabolism* 18, no. 8 (2005): 729, 733.

9. Consortium on the Management of Disorders of Sex Development, *Clinical Guidelines for the Management of Disorders of Sex Development in Childhood* (Intersex Society of North America, 2006), https://dsdguidelines.org/htdocs/clinical, 28; and Consortium on the Management of Disorders of Sex Development, *Handbook for Parents* (Intersex Society of North America, 2006), https://dsdguidelines.org/htdocs/parents, 49–50. I am credited as a contributor to the *Handbook for Parents* because I provided photographs and a biographical note for inclusion (109); I did not coauthor any terminology or recommendations in the handbooks.

10. Alice Dreger, email message to DSD Consortium members, November 22, 2005, received by the author.

11. Eric Vilain et al., "We Used to Call Them Hermaphrodites," *Genetics in Medicine* 9, no. 2 (2007): 65–66.

12. Barbara Thomas, "Report to AISSG on Chicago Consensus Conference October 2005," Androgen Insensitivity Syndrome Support Group, June 2006, https://web.archive.org/web/20180318023840/http://www.aissg.org/PDFs/Barbara-Chicago-Rpt.pdf, 3.

13. Cheryl Chase quoted in Davis, *Contesting Intersex*, 45.

14. I. A. Hughes et al., "Consensus Statement on Management of Intersex Disorders," *Journal of Pediatric Urology* 2, no. 3 (2006): 149.

15. Vilain et al., "We Used to Call Them Hermaphrodites," 66; Hughes et al., "Consensus Statement," *Pediatric Urology*, 149.

16. Consortium on the Management of Disorders of Sex Development, *Clinical Guidelines*, 16; Hughes et al., "Consensus Statement," *Pediatric Urology*, 149.

17. Vilain et al., "We Used to Call Them Hermaphrodites," 66.

18. The full statement was published in three journals: the *Journal of Pediatric Urology*, as cited previously, *Archives of Disease in Childhood*, and

Pediatrics. In addition, a summary was published in the latter. A slightly simplified version by two of the lead authors was published later in *Sexual Development.* See Hughes, Houk, et al., "Consensus Statement on Management of Intersex Disorders," *Archives of Disease in Childhood*; Peter A. Lee, Christopher P. Houk, et al., "Consensus Statement on Management of Intersex Disorders," *Pediatrics* 118, no. 2 (2006): e488–e500; Christopher P. Houk et al., "Summary of Consensus Statement on Intersex Disorders and Their Management," *Pediatrics* 118, no. 2 (2006): 753–57; Christopher P. Houk and Peter A. Lee, "Consensus Statement on Terminology and Management: Disorders of Sex Development," *Sexual Development* 2, nos. 4–5 (2008): 172–80.

19. Vickie Pasterski, Philippa Prentice, et al., "Consequences of the Chicago Consensus on Disorders of Sex Development (DSD): Current Practices in Europe," *Archives of Disease in Childhood* 95, no. 8 (2010): 621. Interestingly, although diagnostic uses of the terms *hermaphrodite* and *pseudohermaphrodite* also reduced over the same period, Pasterski and coauthors report that they fell only 12 percent on average (621).

20. Both handbooks included a statement from three contributors—David Cameron, Esther Morris Leidolf, and Peter Trinkl—that they "would like to make it known that they do not support the term 'Disorders of Sex Development.'" Consortium on the Management of Disorders of Sex Development, *Clinical Guidelines*, ii; and Consortium on the Management of Disorders of Sex Development, *Handbook for Parents*, ii.

21. For example, Elizabeth Reis proposed *divergence of sex development*; Ian Aaronson and Alistair Aaronson proposed *discordant sex development*; Lih-Mei Liao and Margaret Simmonds proposed *diverse sex development*; and Margaret Simmonds separately proposed *variations of reproductive development.* Milton Diamond and Hazel Beh proposed *variations of sex development* and then *differences of sex development.* The version of the consensus statement that appeared in *Sexual Development* acknowledged the emerging debate over terminology. See Elizabeth Reis, "Divergence or Disorder? The Politics of Naming Intersex," *Perspectives in Biology and Medicine* 50, no. 4 (2007): 541; Ian A. Aaronson and Alistair J. Aaronson, "How Should We Classify Intersex Disorders?," *Journal of Pediatric Urology* 6, no. 5 (2010): 444; Lih-Mei Liao and Margaret Simmonds, "A Values-Driven and

Evidence-Based Health Care Psychology for Diverse Sex Development," *Psychology and Sexuality* 5, no. 1 (2014): 85; Margaret Simmonds, "Was 'Variations of Reproductive' Development Considered?" (letter), *Archives of Disease in Childhood*, August 17, 2006, https://web.archive.org/web/20150514044052/http://adc.bmj.com /content/91/7/554/reply; Beh and Diamond, "Variations of Sex Development Instead of Disorders of Sex Development"; Milton Diamond and Hazel G. Beh, "Changes in the Management of Children with Intersex Conditions," *Nature Clinical Practice Endocrinology and Metabolism* 4, no. 1 (2008): 5; Houk and Lee, "Consensus Statement," 173–74.

22. For example, David Cameron, "Re: Variations of Sex Development Instead of Disorders of Sex Development" (letter), *Archives of Disease in Childhood*, August 2, 2006, https://web.archive.org/web /20150514044052/http://adc.bmj.com/content/91/7/554/reply; Holmes, "The Intersex Enchiridion," 388–89; and Viloria, "Promoting Health and Social Progress by Accepting and Depathologizing Benign Intersex Traits," 116.

23. For example, Susannah Cornwall uses a mixture of *intersex* and *intersex/DSD*; Claudia Wiesemann and colleagues alternate between *differences of sex development* (*DSD*)/*intersex* and *intersex/DSD*; and Faisal Ahmed and Martina Rodie suggest that the term *DSD* "can be used to cover both differences and disorders of sex development." See Susannah Cornwall, *Sex and Uncertainty in the Body of Christ: Intersex Conditions and Christian Theology* (Equinox, 2010), 18; Wiesemann et al., "Ethical Principles and Recommendations for the Medical Management of Differences of Sex Development," 671; S. Faisal Ahmed and Martina Rodie, "Investigation and Initial Management of Ambiguous Genitalia," *Best Practice & Research Clinical Endocrinology & Metabolism* 24, no. 2 (2010): 198.

24. Cheryl Chase, "Disorders of Sex Development Similar to More Familiar Disorders" (letter), *Archives of Disease in Childhood*, August 22, 2006, https://web.archive.org/web/20150514044052/http://adc.bmj.com /content/91/7/554/reply.

25. Dreger, Chase, et al., "Changing the Nomenclature/Taxonomy for Intersex," 732.

26. Ellen K. Feder and Katrina Karkazis, "What's in a Name? The Controversy Over 'Disorders of Sex Development,'" *Hastings Center Report* 38, no. 5 (2008): 33.

27. Dreger and Herndon, "Progress and Politics in the Intersex Rights Movement," 208.

28. Vilain et al., "We Used to Call Them Hermaphrodites," 66.

29. Feder and Karkazis, "What's in a Name?," 34–35.

30. Vilain et al., "We Used to Call Them Hermaphrodites," 66.

31. Anonymous support-group member quoted in Simmonds, "Was 'Variations of Reproductive Development' Considered?"; Marie-Noëlle Baechler, "Children Are Not Disorders" (letter), *Archives of Disease in Childhood*, August 29, 2006, https://web.archive.org/web/20150514044052/http://adc.bmj.com/content/91/7/554/reply.

32. Cameron, "Re: Variations of Sex Development Instead of Disorders of Sex Development."

33. Dreger, Chase, et al., "Changing the Nomenclature/Taxonomy," 733.

34. Lynnell Stephani Long, "DSD vs Intersex" (letter), *Archives of Disease in Childhood*, August 23, 2006, https://web.archive.org/web/20150514044052/http://adc.bmj.com/content/91/7/554/reply. Long adds that although "I was, and am, proud to be Intersex," it can be tactically useful to engage doctors "at their own level by using simple medical terminology like DSD."

35. Diamond and Beh, "Changes in the Management of Children with Intersex Conditions," 5, emphasis added.

36. Ellen Feder suggests that the assumption "that there are such things as 'intersexuals'" renders "the characterization of the condition as a disorder offensive." See Feder, "Imperatives of Normality," 226. My argument is different. I think there exist two separate criticisms—one against the construction of disordered people, another against the construction of a medical condition in place of the identity *intersex*. These criticisms imply two different relationships between diagnostic language and identity.

37. Mark Norris Lance and Alessandra Tanesini, "Identity Judgements, Queer Politics" (2000), in *Queer Theory*, ed. Morland and Willox, 178–79.

38. Beh and Diamond, "Variations of Sex Development Instead of Disorders of Sex Development."

39. Feder, "Imperatives of Normality," 226.

40. Hughes et al., "Consensus Statement," *Pediatric Urology*, 155. This is a long-standing tenet of the sociology of medicine—for example, in Mildred Blaxter's classic paper "The Causes of Disease: Women Talking," *Social Science and Medicine* 17, no. 2 (1983): 67.

41. Ralf Werner et al., "46,XY Disorders of Sex Development—the Undermasculinised Male with Disorders of Androgen Action," *Best Practice & Research Clinical Endocrinology & Metabolism* 24, no. 2 (2010): 272; Wilcox and Ransley, "Medicolegal Aspects of Hypospadias," 330; Catherine L. Minto et al., "The Effect of Clitoral Surgery on Sexual Outcome in Individuals Who Have Intersex Conditions with Ambiguous Genitalia: A Cross-Sectional Study," *Lancet* 361, no. 9365 (2003): 1256–57.

42. Hughes et al., "Consensus Statement," *Pediatric Urology*, 150. The handbook for clinicians that appeared in the same year was more circumspect about the benefits of multidisciplinary collaboration, noting that "a dedicated multidisciplinary team is neither a guarantor of nor a necessity of patient-centered care for DSDs." See Consortium on the Management of Disorders of Sex Development, *Clinical Guidelines*, 1.

43. Hughes et al., "Consensus Statement," *Pediatric Urology*, 151, 150.

44. Davis, *Contesting Intersex*, 77, 85–86, 120.

45. For example, Holmes, "Intersex Enchiridion," 404; Alyson K. Spurgas, "(Un)Queering Identity: The Biosocial Production of Intersex/DSD," in *Critical Intersex*, ed. Holmes, 103.

46. Hughes et al., "Consensus Statement," *Pediatric Urology*, 158, 151.

47. Lee, Nordenström, et al., "Global Disorders of Sex Development Update Since 2006," 170.

48. Hughes et al., "Consensus Statement," *Pediatric Urology*, 149. The statement gives examples of specific diagnoses "based on descriptive terms" in table 2 on page 150.

49. Hughes et al., "Consensus Statement," *Pediatric Urology*, 151, 152.

50. Karl Marx, *Capital: A Critical Analysis of Capitalist Production*, vol. 1 (1867), ed. Frederick Engels, trans. Samuel Moore and Edward Aveling (Progress, 1971), 320.

51. Hughes et al., "Consensus Statement," *Pediatric Urology*, 154; Ieuan A. Hughes, "Disorders of Sex Development: A New Definition and

Classification," *Best Practice & Research Clinical Endocrinology & Metabolism* 22, no. 1 (2008): 129.

52. Caroline E. Brain et al., "Holistic Management of DSD," *Best Practice & Research Clinical Endocrinology & Metabolism* 24, no. 2 (2010): 342.

53. Lee, Nordenström, et al., "Global Disorders of Sex Development Update Since 2006," 167.

54. Liao and Simmonds, "A Values-Driven and Evidence-Based Health Care Psychology for Intersex/Diverse Sex Development," 84, 86; Katrina Roen and Vickie Pasterski, "Psychological Research and Intersex/DSD: Recent Developments and Future Directions," *Psychology and Sexuality* 5, no. 1 (2014): 105.

55. Butler, *Gender Trouble*, 190–91.

56. Dreger, "Intersex and Human Rights," 81.

57. Carpenter, "The Human Rights of Intersex People," 77.

58. Lee, Wisniewski, et al., "Advances in Diagnosis and Care of Persons with DSD Over the Last Decade," 4.

59. For the challenge, see Alice Domurat Dreger and Ellen K. Feder, "Still Ignoring Human Rights in Intersex Care" (letter), *Journal of Pediatric Urology* 12, no. 6 (2016): 436; for the response, see Pierre D. E. Mouriquand and Anthony C. Caldamone, "Response to 'Re. Surgery in Disorders of Sex Development (DSD) with a Gender Issue: If (Why), When and How?'" (letter), *Journal of Pediatric Urology* 12, no. 6 (2016): 438.

60. Carpenter, "Human Rights of Intersex People," 76.

61. Roen, "'But We Have to *Do Something*,'" 52; M. DiSandro et al., "Review of Current Surgical Techniques and Medical Management Considerations in the Treatment of Pediatric Patients with Disorders of Sex Development," *Hormone and Metabolic Research* 47, no. 5 (2015): 321.

62. Feder, *Making Sense of Intersex*, 149–50.

63. Mouriquand and Caldamone, "Response to 'Re. Surgery in Disorders of Sex Development,'" 438.

64. Julie Alderson and Naomi Crouch, "Re: Parental Choice on Normalising Cosmetic Genital Surgery" (letter), *British Medical Journal*, October 2, 2015, https://www.bmj.com/content/351/bmj.h5124/rapid-responses.

65. Hughes et al., "Consensus Statement," *Pediatric Urology*, 159.
66. Holmes, "Intersex Enchiridion," 395, emphasis in original.
67. Peter A. Lee and Christopher P. Houk, "The Role of Support Groups, Advocacy Groups, and Other Interested Parties in Improving the Care of Patients with Congenital Adrenal Hyperplasia: Pleas and Warnings," *International Journal of Pediatric Endocrinology* 2010: art. 563640, https://doi.org/10.1155/2010/563640, 4.
68. Ahmed, Achermann, et al., "UK Guidance on the Initial Evaluation of an Infant or an Adolescent with a Suspected Disorder of Sex Development," 14.
69. Marx, *Capital*, 314.
70. Quoted in Melissa Hendricks, "Into the Hands of Babes," *Johns Hopkins Magazine*, September 2000.
71. Vilain et al., "We Used to Call Them Hermaphrodites," 66. Grumbach was also a coauthor of the 2006 policy statement.
72. Ahmed, Gardner, et al., "Management of Children with Disorders of Sex Development," 11.
73. Victoria Grace, *Baudrillard's Challenge: A Feminist Reading* (Routledge, 2000), 21.
74. Mouriquand, Gorduza, et al., "Surgery in Disorders of Sex Development (DSD) with a Gender Issue," 142. Eight coauthors of this paper also contributed to the 2006 policy statement.
75. Alderson et al., "Why Do Parents Recommend Clitoral Surgery?," 56.
76. Sharon E. Preves, "Intersex Narratives: Gender, Medicine, and Identity," in *Sex, Gender, and Sexuality: The New Basics*, ed. Abby L. Ferber et al. (Oxford University Press, 2009), 41.
77. Lee and Houk, "Role of Support Groups," 4.
78. Holmes, *Intersex*, 144.
79. Holmes, *Intersex*, 144.
80. Lee and Houk, "Role of Support Groups," 1–4.
81. To support their position, Lee and Houk note that "recall of specifics from early childhood traumatic situations may be inaccurate," but they do not acknowledge that the "traumatic situations" to which they refer are experiences of medical treatment. See Lee and Houk, "Role of Support Groups," 3.

82. Fredric Jameson, *The Seeds of Time* (Columbia University Press, 1994), 16.

83. Mark Woodward quoted in Kleeman, "'We Don't Know if Your Baby's a Boy or a Girl.'" Valentino Vecchietti has likened such rhetoric to saying, "I need to keep amputating people's feet, I don't want to stop doing it in case I lose the ability to needlessly amputate people's feet, so I must keep doing it." Quoted in Monro et al., *Intersex, Variations of Sex Characteristics, and DSD*, 17.

AFTERWORD: RESISTING MEDICAL NECESSITY

1. Celeste E. Orr, "Covid and Intersex: In/Essential Medical Management," in *Covid and . . .: How to Do Rhetoric in a Pandemic*, ed. Emily Winderman et al. (Michigan State University Press, 2023), 148–49.

2. Hedi L. Claahsen-van der Grinten et al., "Congenital Adrenal Hyperplasia: Current Insights in Pathophysiology, Diagnostics, and Management," *Endocrine Reviews* 43, no. 1 (2022): 94, 116. Strictly speaking, it is dihydrotestosterone that causes the clitoral growth.

3. See, respectively, Gesetz zum Schutz von Kindern mit Varianten der Geschlechtsentwicklung (BGBL I/1082/2021); Μεταρρυθμίσεις στην ιατρικώς υποβοηθούμενη αναπαραγωγή και άλλες επείγουσες ρυθμίσεις (4958/2022); Lög um breytingu á lögum um kynrænt sjálfræði 80/2019 (ódæmigerð kyneinkenni) (154/2020); Gender Identity, Gender Expression, and Sex Characteristics Act (XI/2015); and Direito à autodeterminação da identidade de género e expressão de género e à proteção das características sexuais de cada pessoa (203/XIII/2018).

4. Crocetti, Berry, et al., "Navigating the Complexities of Adult Healthcare for Individuals with Variations of Sex Characteristics," 333.

5. Garland and Travis, *Intersex Embodiment*, 131–37.

6. Morgan Carpenter, "Fixing Bodies and Shaping Narratives: Epistemic Injustice and the Responses of Medicine and Bioethics to Intersex Human Rights Demands," *Clinical Ethics* 19, no. 1 (2024): 6; Matthew Smith, "Where in the World Are Men Most Likely to Sit Down to Wee?," YouGov UK, May 16, 2023, https://yougov.co.uk/society /articles/45713-where-world-are-men-most-likely-sit-down-wee.

7. Peter A. Lee and Christopher P. Houk, "Review of Outcome Information in 46,XX Patients with Congenital Adrenal Hyperplasia Assigned/Reared Male: What Does It Say About Gender Assignment?," *International Journal of Pediatric Endocrinology* 2010: art. 982025, https://doi.org/10.1155/2010/982025, 2.

8. Limor Meoded Danon et al., "Opportunities and Challenges with the German Act for the Protection of Children with Variations of Sex Development," *International Journal of Impotence Research* 35, no. 1 (2023): 39–40.

9. Breen and Roen, "The Rights of Intersex Children in Aotearoa New Zealand," 552, 554.

10. Quoted in Swarr, *Envisioning African Intersex*, 155.

11. Heino F. L. Meyer-Bahlburg, "Censoring Intersex Science: A Medical School Scandal," *Archives of Sexual Behavior* 52, no. 1 (2023): 22.

12. Griffiths, "Queering the Moment of Hypospadias 'Repair,'" 510–11.

13. For example, despite being skeptical of the "supposed medical problems" that doctors cite to justify interventions, Celeste Orr retains a notion of "health problems or body–mind impairments" caused by intersex, for which individuals may "require" care. See Orr, *Cripping Intersex*, 40–41.

BIBLIOGRAPHY

Aaronson, Ian A., and Alistair J. Aaronson. "How Should We Classify Intersex Disorders?" *Journal of Pediatric Urology* 6, no. 5 (2010): 443–46.

Abraham, Nicolas. "Notes on the Phantom: A Complement to Freud's Metapsychology" (1975). In Abraham and Torok, *The Shell and the Kernel*.

Abraham, Nicolas. "Seminar on Dual Unity and the Phantom" (1978). Translated by Tom Goodwin. *Diacritics* 44, no. 4 (2016): 14–39.

Abraham, Nicolas, and Maria Torok. "'The Lost Object—Me': Notes on Endocryptic Identification" (1975). In Abraham and Torok, *The Shell and the Kernel*.

Abraham, Nicolas, and Maria Torok. *The Shell and the Kernel: Renewals of Psychoanalysis*. Edited and translated by Nicholas T. Rand. University of Chicago Press, 1994.

Adorno, Theodor W. *Prisms* (1955). Translated by Samuel Weber and Shierry Weber. Neville Spearman, 1967.

Ahmed, S. Faisal, Carlo Acerini, Tim Cheetham, Justin Davies, Ieuan A. Hughes, Jeremy Kirk, et al. "Re: Parental Choice on Normalising Cosmetic Genital Surgery" (letter). *British Medical Journal*, October 8, 2015. https://www.bmj.com/content/351/bmj.h5124/rr-2.

Ahmed, S. Faisal, John C. Achermann, Wiebke Arlt, Adam H. Balen, Gerry Conway, Zoe L. Edwards, et al. "UK Guidance on the Initial Evaluation of an Infant or an Adolescent with a Suspected Disorder of Sex Development." *Clinical Endocrinology* 75, no. 1 (2011): 12–26.

Ahmed, S. Faisal, Melissa Gardner, and David E. Sandberg. "Management of Children with Disorders of Sex Development: New Care Standards Explained." *Psychology and Sexuality* 5, no. 1 (2014): 5–14.

Ahmed, S. Faisal, and Martina Rodie. "Investigation and Initial Management of Ambiguous Genitalia." *Best Practice & Research Clinical Endocrinology & Metabolism* 24, no. 2 (2010): 197–218.

Ahmed, Sara. *The Cultural Politics of Emotion*. Edinburgh University Press, 2004.

Alderson, Julie, and Naomi Crouch. "Re: Parental Choice on Normalising Cosmetic Genital Surgery" (letter). *British Medical Journal*, October 2, 2015. https://www.bmj.com/content/351/bmj.h5124/rapid -responses.

Alderson, Julie, Mars Skae, and Elizabeth C. Crowne. "Why Do Parents Recommend Clitoral Surgery? Parental Perception of the Necessity, Benefit, and Cost of Early Childhood Clitoral Surgery for Congenital Adrenal Hyperplasia (CAH)." *International Journal of Impotence Research* 35, no. 1 (2023): 56–60.

Alexander, Tamara. "The Medical Management of Intersexed Children: An Analogue for Childhood Sexual Abuse." Intersex Society of North America, 1997. https://isna.org/articles/analog.

Ali, Mostafa M., Mamdouh M. El-Hawy, Ehab M. Galal, Ehab R. Tawfiek, and Ahmed Z. Anwar. "Results of Two-Stage Transverse Preputial Island Flap Urethroplasty for Proximal Hypospadias with Chordee That Mandate Division of the Urethral Plate." *Central European Journal of Urology* 74, no. 1 (2021): 89–94.

Althusser, Louis. "Ideology and Ideological State Apparatuses (Notes Towards an Investigation)" (1970). In *Lenin and Philosophy, and Other Essays*, translated by Ben Brewster. NLB, 1971.

Appiah, K. Anthony. "Identity, Authenticity, Survival: Multicultural Societies and Social Reproduction." In *Multiculturalism: Examining the Politics of Recognition*, edited by Amy Gutmann. Princeton University Press, 1994.

Auchus, Richard J., Selma Feldman Witchel, Kelly R. Leight, Javier Aisenberg, Ricardo Azziz, Tânia A. Bachega, et al. "Guidelines for the Development of Comprehensive Care Centers for Congenital Adrenal Hyperplasia: Guidance from the CARES Foundation Initiative."

International Journal of Pediatric Endocrinology 2010: art. 275213. https://doi.org/10.1155/2010/275213.

Baechler, Marie-Noëlle. "Children Are Not Disorders" (letter). *Archives of Disease in Childhood*, August 29, 2006. https://web.archive.org/web/20150514044052/http://adc.bmj.com/content/91/7/554/reply.

Bailez, M. M., John P. Gearhart, Claude Migeon, and John Rock. "Vaginal Reconstruction After Initial Construction of the External Genitalia in Girls with Salt-Wasting Adrenal Hyperplasia." *Journal of Urology* 148, no. 2 (1992): 680–84.

Bastiaansen, J. A. C. J., M. Thioux, and C. Keysers. "Evidence for Mirror Systems in Emotions." *Philosophical Transactions of the Royal Society of London, B: Biological Sciences* 364, no. 1528 (2009): 2391–404.

Bauman, Zygmunt. *Liquid Modernity.* Polity, 2000.

Beh, Hazel Glenn, and Milton Diamond. "David Reimer's Legacy: Limiting Parental Discretion." *Cardozo Journal of Law and Gender* 12, no. 1 (2005): 5–30.

Bem, Sandra Lipsitz. "Dismantling Gender Polarization and Compulsory Heterosexuality: Should We Turn the Volume Down or Up?" *Journal of Sex Research* 32, no. 4 (1995): 329–34.

Bentwich, Miriam. "On the Inseparability of Gender Eugenics, Ethics, and Public Policy: An Israeli Perspective." *American Journal of Bioethics* 13, no. 10 (2013): 43–45.

Berlant, Lauren. "'68 or The Revolution of Little Queers." In *Feminism Beside Itself,* edited by Diane Elam and Robyn Wiegman. Routledge, 1995.

Berlant, Lauren. "Compassion (and Withholding)." In Berlant, ed., *Compassion.*

Berlant, Lauren, ed. *Compassion: The Culture and Politics of an Emotion.* Routledge, 2004.

Berlant, Lauren. "The Subject of True Feeling: Pain, Privacy, and Politics." In *Cultural Pluralism, Identity Politics, and the Law,* edited by Austin Sarat and Thomas R. Kearns. University of Michigan Press, 1999.

Berlant, Lauren, and Elizabeth Freeman. "Queer Nationality." In Lauren Berlant, *The Queen of America Goes to Washington City: Essays on Sex and Citizenship.* Duke University Press, 1997.

Berlant, Lauren, and Michael Warner. "Sex in Public" (1998). In Michael Warner, *Publics and Counterpublics.* Zone, 2002.

Bersani, Leo. *Homos.* Harvard University Press, 1995.

Bersani, Leo. "Is the Rectum a Grave?" In *AIDS: Cultural Analysis, Cultural Activism*, edited by Douglas Crimp. MIT Press, 1988.

Bird, Jo. "Outside the Law: Intersex, Medicine, and the Discourse of Rights." *Cardozo Journal of Law and Gender* 12, no. 1 (2005): 65–80.

Blasius, Mark. *Gay and Lesbian Politics: Sexuality and the Emergence of a New Ethic*. Temple University Press, 1994.

Blaxter, Mildred. "The Causes of Disease: Women Talking." *Social Science and Medicine* 17, no. 2 (1983): 59–69.

Blum, Harold P. "Separation-Individuation Theory and Attachment Theory." *Journal of the American Psychoanalytic Association* 52, no. 2 (2004): 535–53.

Bowlby, John. *The Making and Breaking of Affectional Bonds*. 1979. Routledge, 2005.

Brain, Caroline E., Sarah M. Creighton, Imran Mushtaq, Polly A. Carmichael, Angela Barnicoat, John W. Honour, et al. "Holistic Management of DSD." *Best Practice & Research Clinical Endocrinology & Metabolism* 24, no. 2 (2010): 335–54.

Breen, Claire, and Katrina Roen. "The Rights of Intersex Children in Aotearoa New Zealand." *International Journal of Children's Rights* 31, no. 3 (2023): 533–67.

Brown, Laura S. *Cultural Competence in Trauma Therapy: Beyond the Flashback*. American Psychological Association, 2008.

Butler, Judith. *Bodies That Matter: On the Discursive Limits of "Sex."* Routledge, 1993.

Butler, Judith. *Gender Trouble: Feminism and the Subversion of Identity*. 2nd ed. Routledge, 2006.

Butler, Judith. *Undoing Gender*. Routledge, 2004.

Byne, William. "Developmental Endocrine Influences on Gender Identity: Implications for Management of Disorders of Sex Development." *Mount Sinai Journal of Medicine* 73, no. 7 (2006): 950–59.

Califia, Patrick (as Pat Califia). "Gay Men, Lesbians, and Sex: Doing It Together" (1983). In Califia, *Public Sex*.

Califia, Patrick (as Pat Califia). "Genderbending: Playing with Roles and Reversals" (1983). In Califia, *Public Sex*.

Califia, Patrick (as Pat Califia). *Public Sex: The Culture of Radical Sex*. 2nd ed. Cleis, 2000.

Califia, Patrick (as Pat Califia). "A Secret Side of Lesbian Sexuality" (1979). In Califia, *Public Sex*.

Cameron, David. "Re: Variations of Sex Development Instead of Disorders of Sex Development" (letter). *Archives of Disease in Childhood*, August 2, 2006. https://web.archive.org/web/20150514044052/http://adc.bmj.com /content/91/7/554/reply.

Carel, Havi. *Phenomenology of Illness*. Oxford University Press, 2016.

Carpenter, Morgan. "Fixing Bodies and Shaping Narratives: Epistemic Injustice and the Responses of Medicine and Bioethics to Intersex Human Rights Demands." *Clinical Ethics* 19, no. 1 (2024): 3–17.

Carpenter, Morgan. "The Human Rights of Intersex People: Addressing Harmful Practices and Rhetoric of Change." *Reproductive Health Matters* 24, no. 47 (2016): 74–84.

Caserio, Robert L. "The Antisocial Thesis in Queer Theory." *PMLA* 121, no. 3 (2006): 819–21.

Chase, Cheryl. "Affronting Reason." In *Looking Queer: Body Image and Identity in Lesbian, Bisexual, Gay, and Transgender Communities*, edited by Dawn Atkins. Harrington Park, 1998.

Chase, Cheryl. "Disorders of Sex Development Similar to More Familiar Disorders" (letter). *Archives of Disease in Childhood*, August 22, 2006. https://web.archive.org/web/20150514044052/http://adc.bmj.com /content/91/7/554/reply.

Chase, Cheryl. "Hermaphrodites with Attitude: Mapping the Emergence of Intersex Political Activism." *GLQ* 4, no. 2 (1998): 189–211.

Chase, Cheryl. "Intersexual Rights" (letter). *Sciences* 33, no. 4 (1993): 3.

Chase, Cheryl. "Re: Measurement of Pudendal Evoked Potentials During Feminizing Genitoplasty: Technique and Applications" (letter). *Journal of Urology* 156, no. 3 (1996): 1139–40.

Chase, Cheryl. "Rethinking Treatment for Ambiguous Genitalia." *Pediatric Nursing* 25, no. 4 (1999): 451–55.

Chase, Cheryl. "What Is the Agenda of the Intersex Patient Advocacy Movement?" *Endocrinologist* 13, no. 3 (2003): 240–42.

Chavhan, Govind B., Dimitri A. Parra, Kamaldine Oudjhane, Stephen F. Miller, Paul S. Babyn, and Joao L. Pippi Salle. "Imaging of Ambiguous Genitalia: Classification and Diagnostic Approach." *RadioGraphics* 28, no. 7 (2008): 1891–904.

Chinn, Sarah E. "Feeling Her Way: Audre Lorde and the Power of Touch."
GLQ 9, nos. 1–2 (2003): 181–204.

Claahsen-van der Grinten, Hedi L., Phyllis W. Speiser, S. Faisal Ahmed,
Wiebke Arlt, Richard J. Auchus, Henrik Falhammar, et al. "Congenital
Adrenal Hyperplasia: Current Insights in Pathophysiology, Diagnostics,
and Management." *Endocrine Reviews* 43, no. 1 (2022): 91–159.

Cloitre, Marylene, Lisa R. Cohen, and Karestan C. Koenen. *Treating Survivors of Childhood Abuse: Psychotherapy for the Interrupted Life*. Guilford,
2006.

Cohen-Kettenis, P. T. "Psychosocial and Psychosexual Aspects of Disorders
of Sex Development." *Best Practice & Research Clinical Endocrinology &
Metabolism* 24, no. 2 (2010): 325–34.

Colapinto, John. *As Nature Made Him: The Boy Who Was Raised as a Girl*.
Quartet, 2000.

Consortium on the Management of Disorders of Sex Development. *Clinical Guidelines for the Management of Disorders of Sex Development in Childhood*. Intersex Society of North America, 2006. https://dsdguidelines
.org/htdocs/clinical.

Consortium on the Management of Disorders of Sex Development. *Handbook for Parents*. Intersex Society of North America, 2006. https://
dsdguidelines.org/htdocs/parents.

Cools, Martine, Anna Nordenström, Ralitsa Robeva, Joanne Hall, Puck
Westerveld, Christa Flück, et al. "Caring for Individuals with a Differ-
ence of Sex Development (DSD): A Consensus Statement." *Nature
Reviews Endocrinology* 14, no. 7 (2018): 415–29.

Coran, Arnold G., and Theodore Z. Polley Jr. "Surgical Management of
Ambiguous Genitalia in the Infant and Child." *Journal of Pediatric Surgery* 26, no. 7 (1991): 812–20.

Cornwall, Susannah. *Sex and Uncertainty in the Body of Christ: Intersex Conditions and Christian Theology*. Equinox, 2010.

Costello, Cary Gabriel. "Beyond Binary Sex and Gender Ideology." In *The
Oxford Handbook of the Sociology of the Body and Embodiment*, edited by
Natalie Boero and Katherine Mason. Oxford University Press, 2020.

Costello, Cary Gabriel. "Understanding Intersex Relationship Issues." In
Expanding the Rainbow: Exploring the Relationships of Bi+, Polyamorous,

Kinky, Ace, Intersex, and Trans People, edited by Brandy L. Simula, J. E. Sumerau, and Andrea Miller. Brill, 2019.

Crawford, Jennifer M., Garry Warne, Sonia Grover, Bridget R. Southwell, and John M. Hutson. "Results from a Pediatric Surgical Centre Justify Early Intervention in Disorders of Sex Development." *Journal of Pediatric Surgery* 44, no. 2 (2009): 413–16.

Creighton, Sarah M. "Surgery for Intersex." *Journal of the Royal Society of Medicine* 94, no. 5 (2001): 218–20.

Creighton, Sarah M., Catherine L. Minto, and Stuart J. Steele. "Objective Cosmetic and Anatomical Outcomes at Adolescence of Feminising Surgery for Ambiguous Genitalia Done in Childhood." *Lancet* 358, no. 9276 (2001): 124–25.

Crimp, Douglas. "Melancholia and Moralism." In *Loss: The Politics of Mourning*, edited by David L. Eng and David Kazanjian. University of California Press, 2002.

Crissman, Halley P., Lauren Warner, Melissa Gardner, Meagan Carr, Aileen Schast, Alexandra L. Quittner, et al. "Children with Disorders of Sex Development: A Qualitative Study of Early Parental Experiences." *International Journal of Pediatric Endocrinology* 2011: art. 10. https://doi.org/10.1186/1687-9856-2011-10.

Crocetti, Daniela, Elia A. G. Arfini, Surya Monro, and Tray Yeadon-Lee. "'You're Basically Calling Doctors Torturers': Stakeholder Framing Issues Around Naming Intersex Rights Claims as Human Rights Abuses." *Sociology of Health & Illness* 42, no. 4 (2020): 943–58.

Crocetti, Daniela, Adeline Berry, and Surya Monro. "Navigating the Complexities of Adult Healthcare for Individuals with Variations of Sex Characteristics: From Paediatric Emergencies to a Sense of Abandonment." *Culture, Health, & Sexuality* 26, no. 3 (2024): 332–45.

Crouch, Naomi S., and Sarah M. Creighton. "Long-Term Functional Outcomes of Female Genital Reconstruction in Childhood." *BJU International* 100, no. 2 (2007): 403–6.

Crouch, Naomi S., Catherine L. Minto, Lih-Mei Liao, Christopher R. J. Woodhouse, and Sarah M. Creighton. "Genital Sensation After Feminizing Genitoplasty for Congenital Adrenal Hyperplasia: A Pilot Study." *BJU International* 93, no. 1 (2004): 135–38.

Crouch, Robert A. "Betwixt and Between: The Past and Future of Inter-sexuality." In Dreger, ed., *Intersex in the Age of Ethics.*

Culbertson, Roberta. "Embodied Memory, Transcendence, and Telling: Recounting Trauma, Re-Establishing the Self." *New Literary History* 26, no. 1 (1995): 169–95.

Cull, Melissa L. "A Support Group's Perspective." *British Medical Journal* 330, no. 7487 (2005): 341–42.

Cvetkovich, Ann. *An Archive of Feelings: Trauma, Sexuality, and Lesbian Public Cultures.* Duke University Press, 2003.

Daaboul, Jorge, and Joel Frader. "Ethics and the Management of the Patient with Intersex: A Middle Way." *Journal of Pediatric Endocrinology and Metabolism* 14, no. 9 (2001): 1575–83.

David. "I Am Not Alone!" *Hermaphrodites with Attitudes*, Winter 1994, 4–5. https://isna.org/files/hwa/winter1995.pdf.

Davis, Georgiann. *Contesting Intersex: The Dubious Diagnosis.* New York University Press, 2015.

Davis, Georgiann. "The Social Costs of Preempting Intersex Traits." *American Journal of Bioethics* 13, no. 10 (2013): 51–53.

Davis, Georgiann, and Erin L. Murphy. "Intersex Bodies as States of Exception: An Empirical Explanation for Unnecessary Surgical Modification." *Feminist Formations* 25, no. 2 (2013): 128–51.

Dayner, Jennifer E., Peter A. Lee, and Christopher P. Houk. "Medical Treatment of Intersex: Parental Perspectives." *Journal of Urology* 172, no. 4 (2004): 1762–65.

Dean, Tim. *Beyond Sexuality.* University of Chicago Press, 2000.

Devore, Tiger (as Howard Devore). "Growing Up in the Surgical Maelstrom." In Dreger, ed., *Intersex in the Age of Ethics.*

DeVun, Leah. *The Shape of Sex: Nonbinary Gender from Genesis to the Renaissance.* Columbia University Press, 2021.

Diamond, Milton. "A Critical Evaluation of the Ontogeny of Human Sexual Behavior." *Quarterly Review of Biology* 40, no. 2 (1965): 147–75.

Diamond, Milton, and Hazel G. Beh. "Changes in the Management of Children with Intersex Conditions." *Nature Clinical Practice Endocrinology & Metabolism* 4, no. 1 (2008): 4–5.

Diamond, Milton, and Jameson Garland. "Evidence Regarding Cosmetic and Medically Unnecessary Surgery on Infants." *Journal of Pediatric Urology* 10, no. 1 (2014): 2–7.

Dinshaw, Carolyn. "Chaucer's Queer Touches/A Queer Touches Chaucer." *Exemplaria* 7, no. 1 (1995): 75–92.

Dinshaw, Carolyn. *Getting Medieval: Sexualities and Communities, Pre- and Postmodern.* Duke University Press, 1999.

Dinshaw, Carolyn, Lee Edelman, Roderick A. Ferguson, Carla Freccero, Elizabeth Freeman, Jack Halberstam (as Judith Halberstam), et al. "Theorizing Queer Temporalities: A Roundtable Discussion." *GLQ* 13, nos. 2–3 (2007): 177–95.

Diprose, Rosalyn. *The Bodies of Women: Ethics, Embodiment, and Sexual Difference.* Routledge, 1994.

DiSandro, M., D. P. Merke, and R. C. Rink. "Review of Current Surgical Techniques and Medical Management Considerations in the Treatment of Pediatric Patients with Disorders of Sex Development." *Hormone and Metabolic Research* 47, no. 5 (2015): 321–28.

Donahoe, Patricia K., D. M. Powell, and M. M. Lee. "Clinical Management of Intersex Abnormalities." *Current Problems in Surgery* 28, no. 8 (1991): 518–79.

Downing, Lisa, Iain Morland, and Nikki Sullivan. *Fuckology: Critical Essays on John Money's Diagnostic Concepts.* University of Chicago Press, 2015.

Dreger, Alice Domurat. "'Ambiguous Sex'—or Ambivalent Medicine? Ethical Issues in the Treatment of Intersexuality." *Hastings Center Report* 28, no. 3 (1998): 24–35.

Dreger, Alice Domurat. *Hermaphrodites and the Medical Invention of Sex.* Harvard University Press, 1998.

Dreger, Alice Domurat. "A History of Intersex: From the Age of Gonads to the Age of Consent." In Dreger, ed., *Intersex in the Age of Ethics.*

Dreger, Alice Domurat. "Intersex and Human Rights: The Long View." In Sytsma, ed., *Ethics and Intersex.*

Dreger, Alice Domurat, ed. *Intersex in the Age of Ethics.* University Publishing Group, 1999.

Dreger, Alice Domurat. "Intersex Treatment as Standard Medical Practice, or, How Wrong I Was." *Medical Humanities Report* 24, no. 3 (2003): 1–4.

Dreger, Alice Domurat. "Jarring Bodies: Thoughts on the Display of Unusual Anatomies." *Perspectives in Biology and Medicine* 43, no. 2 (2000): 161–72.

Dreger, Alice Domurat. "Shifting the Paradigm of Intersex Treatment." Intersex Society of North America, 2003. https://isna.org/compare.

Dreger, Alice Domurat, Cheryl Chase, Aron Sousa, Philip A. Gruppuso, and Joel Frader. "Changing the Nomenclature/Taxonomy for Intersex: A Scientific and Clinical Rationale." *Journal of Pediatric Endocrinology and Metabolism* 18, no. 8 (2005): 729–33.

Dreger, Alice Domurat, and Ellen K. Feder. "Still Ignoring Human Rights in Intersex Care" (letter). *Journal of Pediatric Urology* 12, no. 6 (2016): 436–37.

Dreger, Alice Domurat, Ellen K. Feder, and Anne Tamar-Mattis. "Prenatal Dexamethasone for Congenital Adrenal Hyperplasia: An Ethics Canary in the Modern Medical Mine." *Bioethical Inquiry* 9, no. 3 (2012): 277–94.

Dreger, Alice Domurat, and April M. Herndon. "Progress and Politics in the Intersex Rights Movement: Feminist Theory in Action." *GLQ* 15, no. 2 (2009): 199–224.

Driver, Betsy. Preface to special issue on intersex. *Cardozo Journal of Law and Gender* 12, no. 1 (2005): 1–3.

Duguid, A., S. Morrison, A. Robertson, J. Chalmers, G. Youngson, and S. F. Ahmed. "The Psychological Impact of Genital Anomalies on the Parents of Affected Children." *Acta Paediatrica* 96, no. 3 (2007): 348–52.

Eckert, Lena. *Intersexualization: The Clinic and the Colony*. Routledge, 2017.

Edelman, Lee. *No Future: Queer Theory and the Death Drive*. Duke University Press, 2004.

Edelman, Lee. "Queer Theory: Unstating Desire." *GLQ* 2, no. 4 (1995): 343–46.

Ehrenreich, Nancy, with Mark Barr. "Intersex Surgery, Female Genital Cutting, and the Selective Condemnation of 'Cultural Practices.'" *Harvard Civil Rights–Civil Liberties Law Review* 40, no. 1 (2005): 71–140.

Ellens, Rebecca E. H., Dana M. Bakula, Alexandria J. Mullins, Kristy J. Scott Reyes, Paul Austin, Laurence Baskin, et al. "Psychological Adjustment of Parents of Children Born with Atypical Genitalia 1 Year After Genitoplasty." *Journal of Urology* 198, no. 4 (2017): 914–20.

English, Deirdre, Amber Hollibaugh, and Gayle Rubin. "Talking Sex: A Conversation on Sexuality and Feminism." *Feminist Review*, no. 11 (1982): 40–51.

Erikson, Kai T. *Everything in Its Path: Destruction of Community in the Buffalo Creek Flood*. Simon and Schuster, 1976.

Eyal, Gil. "Identity and Trauma: Two Forms of the Will to Memory." *History and Memory* 16, no. 1 (2004): 5–36.

Farhat, Walid A. "Early Intervention of CAH Surgical Management." *Journal of Pediatric and Adolescent Gynecology* 18, no. 1 (2005): 66–69.

Farkas, A., B. Chertin, and I. Hadas-Halpren. "1-Stage Feminizing Genitoplasty: 8 Years of Experience with 49 Cases." *Journal of Urology* 165, no. 6 (2001): 2341–46.

Fausto-Sterling, Anne. "The Five Sexes: Why Male and Female Are Not Enough." *Sciences* 33, no. 2 (1993): 20–25.

Fausto-Sterling, Anne. *Myths of Gender: Biological Theories About Women and Men*. Basic, 1985.

Fausto-Sterling, Anne. *Sexing the Body: Gender Politics and the Construction of Sexuality*. Basic, 2000.

Feder, Ellen K. "Doctor's Orders: Parents and Intersexed Children." In *The Subject of Care: Feminist Perspectives on Dependency*, edited by Eva Feder Kittay and Ellen K. Feder. Rowman and Littlefield, 2002.

Feder, Ellen K. "Imperatives of Normality: From 'Intersex' to 'Disorders of Sex Development.'" *GLQ* 15, no. 2 (2009): 225–47.

Feder, Ellen K. *Making Sense of Intersex: Changing Ethical Perspectives in Biomedicine*. Indiana University Press, 2014.

Feder, Ellen K., and Katrina Karkazis. "What's in a Name? The Controversy Over 'Disorders of Sex Development.'" *Hastings Center Report* 38, no. 5 (2008): 33–36.

Fénichel, Patrick, Françoise Paris, Pascal Philibert, Sylvie Hiéronimus, Laura Gaspari, Jean-Yves Kurzenne, et al. "Molecular Diagnosis of 5α-Reductase Deficiency in 4 Elite Young Female Athletes Through Hormonal Screening for Hyperandrogenism." *Journal of Clinical Endocrinology and Metabolism* 98, no. 6 (2013): e1055–59.

Fivush, Robyn, and Katherine Nelson. "Culture and Language in the Emergence of Autobiographical Memory." *Psychological Science* 15, no. 9 (2004): 573–77.

Foster, Hal. "Death in America." *October*, no. 75 (1996): 37–60.

Foucault, Michel. "Body/Power" (1975). Interview by editorial collective of *Quel Corps?* In Foucault, *Power/Knowledge*.

Foucault, Michel. "Powers and Strategies" (1977). Interview by Jean Borreil, Geneviève Fraisse, Jacques Rancière, Pierre Saint-Germain, Michel Souletie, Patrick Vauday, et al. In Foucault, *Power/Knowledge*.

Foucault, Michel. *Power/Knowledge: Selected Interviews and Other Writings, 1972–1977*. Edited and translated by Colin Gordon. Pantheon, 1980.

Foucault, Michel. "Prison Talk" (1975). Interview by Jean-Jacques Brochier. In Foucault, *Power/Knowledge*.

Foucault, Michel. "Sex, Power, and the Politics of Identity" (1984). Interview by B. Gallagher and A. Wilson. In *Ethics: Subjectivity and Truth*, vol. 1 of *The Essential Works of Foucault, 1954–1984*, edited by Paul Rabinow and translated by Robert Hurley et al. New Press, 1997.

Foucault, Michel. *The Will to Knowledge*. Vol. 1 of *The History of Sexuality* (1976). Translated by Robert Hurley. Penguin, 1978.

Frank, Arthur W. *The Wounded Storyteller: Body, Illness, and Ethics*. University of Chicago Press, 1995.

Fraser, Nancy. "Rethinking the Public Sphere: A Contribution to the Critique of Actually Existing Democracy." In *Habermas and the Public Sphere*, edited by Craig Calhoun. MIT Press, 1992.

Freeman, Elizabeth. "Packing History, Count(er)ing Generations." *New Literary History* 31, no. 4 (2000): 727–44.

Freeman, Elizabeth. "Time Binds, or, Erotohistoriography." *Social Text* 23, nos. 3–4 (2005): 57–68.

Freud, Sigmund. "Analyse der Phobie eines fünfjährigen Knaben." In *Gesammelte Werke*, vol. 7. Imago, 1941.

Freud, Sigmund. *On the History of the Psycho-Analytic Movement, Papers on Metapsychology, and Other Works*. Vol. 14 of *The Standard Edition of the Complete Psychological Works of Sigmund Freud*. Edited and translated by James Strachey. Hogarth, 1957.

Freud, Sigmund. "Repression" (1915). In Freud, *On the History of the Psycho-Analytic Movement*.

Freud, Sigmund. "The Unconscious" (1915). In Freud, *On the History of the Psycho-Analytic Movement*.

Friedman, Asia. *Blind to Sameness: Sexpectations and the Social Construction of Male and Female Bodies*. University of Chicago Press, 2013.

Garland, Caroline, ed. *Understanding Trauma: A Psychoanalytical Approach.* Duckworth, 1998.

Garland, Fae, and Mitchell Travis. *Intersex Embodiment: Legal Frameworks Beyond Identity and Disorder.* Bristol University Press, 2023.

Garland, Fae, and Mitchell Travis. "Temporal Bodies: Emergencies, Emergence, and Intersex Embodiment." In *A Jurisprudence of the Body*, edited by Chris Dietz, Mitchell Travis, and Michael Thomson. Palgrave Macmillan, 2020.

Gearhart, J. P., A. Burnett, and J. H. Owen. "In Reply: Re: Measurement of Pudendal Evoked Potentials During Feminizing Genitoplasty: Technique and Applications" (letter). *Journal of Urology* 156, no. 3 (1996): 1140.

Gill-Peterson, Jules (as Julian Gill-Peterson). *Histories of the Transgender Child.* University of Minnesota Press, 2018.

Goss, Katie. "Intersex's New Materialism: More-Than-Binary Bio-Logics in Lucia Puenzo's *XXY.*" *Transgender Studies Quarterly* 9, no. 2 (2022): 228–47.

Grabham, Emily. "Bodily Integrity and the Surgical Management of Intersex." *Body & Society* 18, no. 2 (2012): 1–26.

Grabham, Emily. "Citizen Bodies, Intersex Citizenship." *Sexualities* 10, no. 1 (2007): 29–48.

Grace, Victoria. *Baudrillard's Challenge: A Feminist Reading.* Routledge, 2000.

Greenberg, Julie A. *Intersexuality and the Law: Why Sex Matters.* New York University Press, 2012.

Griffiths, David Andrew. "Queering the Moment of Hypospadias 'Repair.'" *GLQ* 27, no. 4 (2021): 499–523.

Griffiths, David Andrew. "Shifting Syndromes: Sex Chromosome Variations and Intersex Classifications." *Social Studies of Science* 48, no. 1 (2018): 125–48.

Grillo, Trina, and Stephanie M. Wildman. "Obscuring the Importance of Race: The Implication of Making Comparisons Between Racism and Sexism (or Other -Isms)." *Duke Law Journal*, no. 2 (1991): 397–412.

Groveman, Sherri A. "The Hanukkah Bush: Ethical Implications in the Clinical Management of Intersex." In Dreger, ed., *Intersex in the Age of Ethics.*

Grover, Sonia R., Chloe A. Hanna, and Michele A. O'Connell. "Introduction: Changing Landscapes." In *Disorders|Differences of Sex Development:*

An Integrated Approach to Management, 2nd ed., edited by John M. Hutson, Sonia R. Grover, Michele A. O'Connell, Aurore Bouty, and Chloe A. Hanna. Springer Nature Singapore, 2020.

Halberstam, Jack (as Judith Halberstam). *In a Queer Time and Place: Transgender Bodies, Subcultural Lives*. New York University Press, 2005.

Halberstam, Jack (as Judith Halberstam). "Lesbian Masculinity, or Even Stone Butches Get the Blues." *Women and Performance* 8, no. 2 (1996): 61–73.

Halley, Janet E. "'Like Race' Arguments." In *What's Left of Theory? New Work on the Politics of Literary Theory*, edited by Judith Butler, John Guillory, and Kendall Thomas. Routledge, 2000.

Halperin, David M. *Saint Foucault: Towards a Gay Hagiography*. Oxford University Press, 1995.

Harrington, Ralph. "On the Tracks of Trauma: Railway Spine Reconsidered." *Journal of the Society for the Social History of Medicine* 16, no. 2 (2003): 209–23.

Hegarty, Peter, and Cheryl Chase. "Intersex Activism, Feminism, and Psychology" (2000). In Morland and Willox, eds., *Queer Theory*.

Hegarty, Peter, Marta Prandelli, Tove Lundberg, Lih-Mei Liao, Sarah Creighton, and Katrina Roen. "Drawing the Line Between Essential and Nonessential Interventions on Intersex Characteristics with European Health Care Professionals." *Review of General Psychology* 25, no. 1 (2021): 101–14.

Hegarty, Peter, and Annette Smith. "Public Understanding of Intersex: An Update on Recent Findings." *International Journal of Impotence Research* 35, no. 1 (2023): 72–77.

Hemesath, Tatiana Prade, Leila Cristina Pedroso de Paula, Clarissa Gutierrez Carvalho, Julio Cesar Loguercio Leite, Guilherme Guaragna-Filho, and Eduardo Corrêa Costa. "Controversies on Timing of Sex Assignment and Surgery in Individuals with Disorders of Sex Development: A Perspective." *Frontiers in Pediatrics* 6 (2019): art. 419. https://doi.org/10.3389/fped.2018.00419.

Hendricks, Melissa. "Into the Hands of Babes." *Johns Hopkins Magazine*, September 2000.

Hendricks, Melissa. "Is It a Boy or a Girl?" *Johns Hopkins Magazine*, November 1993.

Hensle, Terry W., Ahmad Shabsigh, Ridwan Shabsigh, Elizabeth A. Reiley, and Heino F. L. Meyer-Bahlburg. "Sexual Function Following Bowel Vaginoplasty." *Journal of Urology* 175, no. 6 (2006): 2283–86.

Hermer, Laura D. "A Moratorium on Intersex Surgeries? Law, Science, Identity, and Bioethics at the Crossroads." *Cardozo Journal of Law and Gender* 13, no. 2 (2007): 255–72.

Hillman, Thea. *Intersex (for Lack of a Better Word).* Manic D Press, 2008.

Hird, Myra J., and Jenz Germon. "The Intersexual Body and the Medical Regulation of Gender." In *Constructing Gendered Bodies*, edited by Kathryn Backett-Milburn and Linda McKie. Palgrave, 2001.

Hollibaugh, Amber. "My Dangerous Desires: Falling in Love with Stone Butches, Passing Women, and Girls (Who Are Guys) Who Catch My Eye" (2000). In *Queer Cultures*, edited by Deborah Carlin and Jennifer DiGrazia. Pearson Prentice Hall, 2004.

Hollway, Wendy. "Theorizing Heterosexuality: A Response." *Feminism & Psychology* 3, no. 3 (1993): 412–17.

Holmes, M. Morgan, ed. *Critical Intersex.* Ashgate, 2009.

Holmes, M. Morgan. "Distracted Attentions: Intersexuality and Human Rights Protections." *Cardozo Journal of Law and Gender* 12, no. 1 (2005): 127–34.

Holmes, M. Morgan. *Intersex: A Perilous Difference.* Susquehanna University Press, 2008.

Holmes, M. Morgan. "The Intersex Enchiridion: Naming and Knowledge." *Somatechnics* 1, no. 2 (2011): 388–411.

Holmes, M. Morgan. "Mind the Gaps: Intersex and (Re-Productive) Spaces in Disability Studies and Bioethics." *Bioethical Inquiry* 5, no. 2 (2008): 169–81.

Holmes, M. Morgan. "Queer Cut Bodies." In *Queer Frontiers: Millennial Geographies, Genders, and Generations*, edited by Joseph A. Boone, Martin Dupuis, Martin Meeker, Karin Quimby, Cindy Sarver, Debra Silverman, et al. University of Wisconsin Press, 2000.

Holmes, M. Morgan. "Queer Cut Bodies: Intersexuality and Homophobia in Medical Practice." University of Southern California, 1995. https://web
.archive.org/web/20060703155923/http://www.usc.edu/libraries
/archives/queerfrontiers/queer/papers/holmes.long.html.

Horkheimer, Max. "Materialism and Morality" (1933). In *Between Philosophy and Social Science: Selected Early Writings*, translated by G. Frederick Hunter, Matthew S. Kramer, and John Torpey. MIT Press, 1993.

Horowitz, Sarah. "The Middle Sex." *San Francisco Weekly*, February 1, 1995.

Houk, Christopher P., Ieuan A. Hughes, S. Faisal Ahmed, Peter A. Lee, and the Writing Committee for the International Intersex Consensus Conference Participants. "Summary of Consensus Statement on Intersex Disorders and Their Management." *Pediatrics* 118, no. 2 (2006): 753–57.

Houk, Christopher P., and Peter A. Lee. "Consensus Statement on Terminology and Management: Disorders of Sex Development." *Sexual Development* 2, nos. 4–5 (2008): 172–80.

Hrabovszky, Zoltan, and John M. Hutson. "Surgical Treatment of Intersex Abnormalities: A Review." *Surgery* 131, no. 1 (2002): 92–104.

Hughes, Ieuan A. "Disorders of Sex Development: A New Definition and Classification." *Best Practice & Research Clinical Endocrinology & Metabolism* 22, no. 1 (2008): 119–34.

Hughes, Ieuan A., Christopher P. Houk, S. Faisal Ahmed, Peter A. Lee, and Lawson Wilkins Pediatric Endocrine Society (LWPES)/European Society for Paediatric Endocrinology (ESPE) Consensus Group. "Consensus Statement on Management of Intersex Disorders." *Archives of Disease in Childhood* 91, no. 7 (2006): 554–63.

Hughes, Ieuan A., Christopher P. Houk, S. Faisal Ahmed, Peter A. Lee, and Lawson Wilkins Pediatric Endocrine Society (LWPES)/European Society for Paediatric Endocrinology (ESPE) Consensus Group. "Consensus Statement on Management of Intersex Disorders." *Journal of Pediatric Urology* 2, no. 3 (2006): 148–62.

Human Rights Watch. *"I Want to Be Like Nature Made Me": Medically Unnecessary Surgeries on Intersex Children in the US*. Human Rights Watch, 2017.

Ingham, Graham. "Mental Work in a Trauma Patient." In Garland, ed., *Understanding Trauma*.

Inter, Laura (pseud.). "Finding My Compass." Translated by Leslie Jaye. *Narrative Inquiry in Bioethics* 5, no. 2 (2015): 95–98.

Intersex Society of North America. "Why Doesn't ISNA Want to Eradicate Gender?" 2006. https://www.isna.org/faq/not_eradicating_gender.

Jameson, Fredric. *The Seeds of Time*. Columbia University Press, 1994.

Joint LWPES/ESPE CAH Working Group. "Consensus Statement on 21-Hydroxylase Deficiency from the Lawson Wilkins Pediatric Endocrine Society and the European Society for Paediatric Endocrinology." *Journal of Clinical Endocrinology and Metabolism* 87, no. 9 (2002): 4048–53.

Jones, Brendan C., Mike O'Brien, Janet Chase, Bridget R. Southwell, and John M. Hutson. "Early Hypospadias Surgery May Lead to a Better Long-Term Psychosexual Outcome." *Journal of Urology* 182, supp. 4 (2009): 1744–50.

Jones, Melinda. "Intersex Genital Mutilation—a Western Version of FGM." *International Journal of Children's Rights* 25, no. 2 (2017): 396–411.

Jordan-Young, Rebecca M. *Brain Storm: The Flaws in the Science of Sex Differences*. Harvard University Press, 2010.

Jürgensen, Martina, Eva Hampel, Olaf Hiort, and Ute Thyen. "'Any Decision Is Better Than None': Decision-Making About Sex of Rearing for Siblings with 17β-Hydroxysteroid-Dehydrogenase-3 Deficiency." *Archives of Sexual Behavior* 35, no. 3 (2006): 359–71.

Karkazis, Katrina. *Fixing Sex: Intersex, Medical Authority, and Lived Experience*. Duke University Press, 2008.

Katz, Pearl. "Ritual in the Operating Room." *Ethnology* 20, no. 4 (1981): 335–50.

Kessler, Suzanne J. *Lessons from the Intersexed*. Rutgers University Press, 1998.

Kessler, Suzanne J. "The Medical Construction of Gender: Case Management of Intersexed Infants." *Signs* 16, no. 1 (1990): 3–26.

Kleeman, Jenny. "'We Don't Know If Your Baby's a Boy or a Girl': Growing Up Intersex." *The Guardian*, July 2, 2016. https://www.theguardian.com/world/2016/jul/02/male-and-female-what-is-it-like-to-be-intersex.

Koyama, Emi. *Intersex Critiques: Notes on Intersex, Disability, and Biomedical Ethics*. Confluere, 2003.

Kyriakou, Andreas, Arianne Dessens, Jillian Bryce, Violeta Iotova, Anders Juul, Maciej Krawczynski, et al. "Current Models of Care for Disorders of Sex Development: Results from an International Survey of Specialist Centres." *Orphanet Journal of Rare Diseases* 11 (2016): art. 155. https://doi.org/10.1186/s13023-016-0534-8.

Lampalzer, Ute, Peer Briken, and Katinka Schweizer. "Dealing with Uncertainty and Lack of Knowledge in Diverse Sex Development: Controversies on Early Surgery and Questions of Consent." *Sexual Medicine* 8, no. 3 (2020): 472–89.

Lance, Mark Norris, and Alessandra Tanesini. "Identity Judgements, Queer Politics" (2000). In Morland and Willox, eds., *Queer Theory*.

Lee, Peter A., and Christopher P. Houk. "Review of Outcome Information in 46,XX Patients with Congenital Adrenal Hyperplasia Assigned/ Reared Male: What Does It Say About Gender Assignment?" *International Journal of Pediatric Endocrinology* 2010: art. 982025. https://doi.org /10.1155/2010/982025.

Lee, Peter A., and Christopher P. Houk. "The Role of Support Groups, Advocacy Groups, and Other Interested Parties in Improving the Care of Patients with Congenital Adrenal Hyperplasia: Pleas and Warnings." *International Journal of Pediatric Endocrinology* 2010: art. 563640. https:// doi.org/10.1155/2010/563640.

Lee, Peter A., Christopher P. Houk, S. Faisal Ahmed, Ieuan A. Hughes, in collaboration with the participants in the International Consensus Conference on Intersex organized by the Lawson Wilkins Pediatric Endocrine Society and the European Society for Paediatric Endocrinology. "Consensus Statement on Management of Intersex Disorders." *Pediatrics* 118, no. 2 (2006): e488–e500.

Lee, Peter A., Anna Nordenström, Christopher P. Houk, S. Faisal Ahmed, Richard Auchus, Arlene Baratz, et al. "Global Disorders of Sex Development Update Since 2006: Perceptions, Approach, and Care." *Hormone Research in Paediatrics* 85, no. 3 (2016): 158–80.

Lee, Peter A., Amy B. Wisniewski, Laurence Baskin, Maria G. Vogiatzi, Eric Vilain, Stephen M. Rosenthal, et al., on behalf of the Drugs and Therapeutics Committee of the Pediatric Endocrine Society. "Advances in Diagnosis and Care of Persons with DSD Over the Last Decade." *International Journal of Pediatric Endocrinology* 2014: art. 19. https://doi .org/10.1186/1687-9856-2014-19.

Leidolf, Esther Morris. "The Missing Vagina Monologue . . . and Beyond." *Journal of Gay and Lesbian Psychotherapy* 10, no. 2 (2006): 77–92.

Lennon, Kathleen. "Making Life Livable: Transsexuality and Bodily Transformation." *Radical Philosophy*, no. 140 (2006): 26–34.

Lev, Arlene Istar. "Intersexuality in the Family: An Unacknowledged Trauma." *Journal of Gay and Lesbian Psychotherapy* 10, no. 2 (2006): 27–56.

Leys, Ruth. *Trauma: A Genealogy.* University of Chicago Press, 2000.

Liao, Lih-Mei. "Learning to Assist Women Born with Atypical Genitalia: Journey Through Ignorance, Taboo, and Dilemma." *Journal of Reproductive and Infant Psychology* 21, no. 3 (2003): 229–38.

Liao, Lih-Mei. "Stonewalling Emotion." *Narrative Inquiry in Bioethics* 5, no. 2 (2015): 143–50.

Liao, Lih-Mei. *Variations in Sex Development: Medicine, Culture, and Psychological Practice.* Cambridge University Press, 2023.

Liao, Lih-Mei, and Katrina Roen. "The Role of Psychologists in Multi-Disciplinary Teams for Intersex/Diverse Sex Development: Interviews with British and Swedish Clinical Specialists." *Psychology and Sexuality* 12, no. 3 (2021): 202–16.

Liao, Lih-Mei, and Margaret Simmonds. "A Values-Driven and Evidence-Based Health Care Psychology for Diverse Sex Development." *Psychology and Sexuality* 5, no. 1 (2014): 83–101.

Lima, Mario, Giovanni Ruggeri, Beatrice Randi, Marcello Dòmini, Tommaso Gargano, Enrico La Pergola, et al. "Vaginal Replacement in the Pediatric Age Group: A 34-Year Experience of Intestinal Vaginoplasty in Children and Young Girls." *Journal of Pediatric Surgery* 45, no. 10 (2010): 2087–91.

Lindemann, Hilde. "The Power of Parents and the Agency of Children." In *Surgically Shaping Children: Technology, Ethics, and the Pursuit of Normality*, edited by Erik Parens. Johns Hopkins University Press, 2006.

Lohman, Eric, and Stephani Lohman. *Raising Rosie: Our Story of Parenting an Intersex Child.* Jessica Kingsley, 2018.

Long, Lynnell Stephani. "DSD vs Intersex" (letter). *Archives of Disease in Childhood*, August 23, 2006. https://web.archive.org/web/20150514044052/http://adc.bmj.com/content/91/7/554/reply.

Love, Heather. *Feeling Backward: Loss and the Politics of Queer History.* Harvard University Press, 2007.

Luckhurst, Roger. "Traumaculture." *New Formations*, no. 50 (2003): 28–47.

Machado, Paula Sandrine, Angelo Brandelli Costa, Henrique Caetano Nardi, Anna Martha Vaitses Fontanari, Igor Rabuske Araujo, and

Daniela Riva Knauth. "Follow-up of Psychological Outcomes of Interventions in Patients Diagnosed with Disorders of Sexual Development: A Systematic Review." *Journal of Health Psychology* 21, no. 10 (2016): 2195–206.

MacKenzie, Drew, Annette Huntington, and Jean A. Gilmour. "The Experiences of People with an Intersex Condition: A Journey from Silence to Voice." *Journal of Clinical Nursing* 18, no. 12 (2009): 1775–83.

Magubane, Zine. "Spectacles and Scholarship: Caster Semenya, Intersex Studies, and the Problem of Race in Feminist Theory." *Signs* 39, no. 3 (2014): 761–85.

Main, Mary, Nancy Kaplan, and Jude Cassidy. "Security in Infancy, Childhood, and Adulthood: A Move to the Level of Representation." *Monographs of the Society for Research in Child Development* 50, nos. 1–2 (1985): 66–104.

Mak, Geertje. *Doubting Sex: Inscriptions, Bodies, and Selves in Nineteenth-Century Hermaphrodite Case Histories.* Manchester University Press, 2012.

Malatino, Hil (as Hilary Malatino). *Queer Embodiment: Monstrosity, Medical Violence, and Intersex Experience.* University of Nebraska Press, 2019.

Marx, Karl. *Capital: A Critical Analysis of Capitalist Production.* Vol. 1 (1867). Edited by Frederick Engels. Translated by Samuel Moore and Edward Aveling. Progress, 1971.

Matsui, Futoshi, Kenji Shimada, Fumi Matsumoto, Toshihiko Itesako, Keigo Nara, Shinobu Ida, et al. "Long-Term Outcome of Ovotesticular Disorder of Sex Development: A Single Center Experience." *International Journal of Urology* 18, no. 3 (2011): 231–36.

McCullough, Laurence B. "Critically Appraising Prenatal Genetic Diagnosis to Prevent Disorders of Sexual Development: An Opportunity Missed." *American Journal of Bioethics* 13, no. 10 (2013): 1–3.

Mediã, Line Merete, Lena Fauske, Solrun Sigurdardottir, Kristin J. Billaud Feragen, Charlotte Heggeli, and Anne Wæhre. "'It Was Supposed to Be a Secret': A Study of Disclosure and Stigma as Experienced by Adults with Differences of Sex Development." *Health Psychology and Behavioral Medicine* 10, no. 1 (2022): 579–95.

Mendonca, Berenice Bilharinho, Sorahia Domenice, Ivo J. P. Arnhold, and Elaine M. F. Costa. "46,XY Disorders of Sex Development (DSD)." *Clinical Endocrinology* 70, no. 2 (2009): 173–87.

Meoded Danon, Limor. "The Body/Secret Dynamic: Life Experiences of Intersexed People in Israel." *SAGE Open* 5, no. 2 (2015). https://doi.org /10.1177/2158244015580370.

Meoded Danon, Limor. "Temporal Sociomedical Approaches to Intersex* Bodies." *History and Philosophy of the Life Sciences* 44 (2022): art. 28. https:// doi.org/10.1007/s40656-022-00511-0.

Meoded Danon, Limor, Katinka Schweizer, and Barbara Thies. "Opportunities and Challenges with the German Act for the Protection of Children with Variations of Sex Development." *International Journal of Impotence Research* 35, no. 1 (2023): 38–45.

Meoded Danon, Limor, and Niza Yanay. "Intersexuality: On Secret Bodies and Secrecy." *Studies in Gender and Sexuality* 17, no. 1 (2016): 57–72.

Merleau-Ponty, Maurice. *The Visible and the Invisible* (1964). Edited by Claude Lefort. Translated by Alphonso Lingis. Northwestern University Press, 1968.

Meyer-Bahlburg, Heino F. L. "Censoring Intersex Science: A Medical School Scandal." *Archives of Sexual Behavior* 52, no. 1 (2023): 21–25.

Meyer-Bahlburg, Heino F. L. "Misrepresentation of Evidence Favoring Early Normalizing Surgery for Atypical Sex Anatomies: Response to Baratz and Feder" (letter). *Archives of Sexual Behavior* 44, no. 7 (2015): 1765–68.

Meyer-Bahlburg, Heino F. L. "The Timing of Genital Surgery in Somatic Intersexuality: Surveys of Patients' Preferences." *Hormone Research in Paediatrics* 95, no. 1 (2022): 12–20.

Michala, Lina, Lih-Mei Liao, Dan Wood, Gerard S. Conway, and Sarah M. Creighton. "Practice Changes in Childhood Surgery for Ambiguous Genitalia?" *Journal of Pediatric Urology* 10, no. 5 (2014): 934–40.

Mieszczak, Jakub, Christopher P. Houk, and Peter A. Lee. "Assignment of the Sex of Rearing in the Neonate with a Disorder of Sex Development." *Current Opinion in Pediatrics* 21, no. 4 (2009): 541–47.

Miller, Walter L., Sharon E. Oberfield, Phyllis W. Speiser, Laurence S. Baskin, Patricia K. Donahoe, Claire Nihoul-Fékété, et al. "Authors' Response: Regarding the Consensus Statement on 21-Hydroxylase Deficiency from the Lawson Wilkins Pediatric Endocrine Society and the

European Society for Paediatric Endocrinology." *Journal of Clinical Endo-crinology and Metabolism* 88, no. 7 (2003): 3454–56.

Minto, Catherine L., Lih-Mei Liao, Christopher R. J. Woodhouse, Phillip G. Ransley, and Sarah M. Creighton. "The Effect of Clitoral Surgery on Sexual Outcome in Individuals Who Have Intersex Conditions with Ambiguous Genitalia: A Cross-Sectional Study." *Lancet* 361, no. 9365 (2003): 1252–57.

Money, John. "Hermaphroditism, Gender, and Precocity in Hyperadrenocorticism: Psychologic Findings." *Bulletin of the Johns Hopkins Hospital* 96, no. 6 (1955): 253–64.

Money, John. *The Psychologic Study of Man*. Charles C. Thomas, 1957.

Money, John. *Sex Errors of the Body: Dilemmas, Education, Counseling*. Johns Hopkins University Press, 1968.

Money, John, and Anke A. Ehrhardt. *Man and Woman, Boy and Girl: The Differentiation and Dimorphism of Gender Identity from Conception to Maturity*. Johns Hopkins University Press, 1972.

Money, John, Joan G. Hampson, and John L. Hampson. "Hermaphroditism: Recommendations Concerning Assignment of Sex, Change of Sex, and Psychologic Management." *Bulletin of the Johns Hopkins Hospital* 97, no. 4 (1955): 284–300.

Monro, Surya, Daniela Crocetti, Tray Yeadon-Lee, Fae Garland, and Mitch Travis. *Intersex, Variations of Sex Characteristics, and DSD: The Need for Change*. University of Huddersfield, 2017.

Montagu, Ashley. *Touching: The Human Significance of the Skin*. Columbia University Press, 1971.

Morland, Iain. "Between Critique and Reform: Ways of Reading the Intersex Controversy." In Holmes, ed., *Critical Intersex*.

Morland, Iain. "Cybernetic Sexology." In Downing, Morland, and Sullivan, *Fuckology*.

Morland, Iain. "Gender, Genitals, and the Meaning of Being Human." In Downing, Morland, and Sullivan, *Fuckology*.

Morland, Iain. "The Injured World: Intersex and the Phenomenology of Feeling." *differences: A Journal of Feminist Cultural Studies* 23, no. 2 (2012): 20–41.

Morland, Iain. "Intersex Surgery Between the Gaze and the Subject." *Transgender Studies Quarterly* 9, no. 2 (2022): 160–71.

Morland, Iain. "Intersex Treatment and the Promise of Trauma." In *Gender and the Science of Difference: Cultural Politics of Contemporary Science and Medicine*, edited by Jill A. Fisher. Rutgers University Press, 2011.

Morland, Iain. "Is Intersexuality Real?" *Textual Practice* 15, no. 3 (2001): 527–47.

Morland, Iain. "What Can Queer Theory Do for Intersex?" *GLQ: A Journal of Lesbian and Gay Studies* 15, no. 2 (2009): 285–312.

Morland, Iain. "Why Five Sexes Are Not Enough." In *The Ashgate Research Companion to Queer Theory*, edited by Noreen Giffney and Michael O'Rourke. Ashgate, 2009.

Morland, Iain, and Annabelle Willox, eds. *Queer Theory*. Palgrave, 2005.

Morris, Esther. "The Self I Will Never Know." *New Internationalist*, January–February 2004, 25–27.

Morton, Donald. "Birth of the Cyberqueer." *PMLA* 110, no. 3 (1995): 369–81.

Mouriquand, Pierre D. E., and Anthony C. Caldamone. "Response to 'Re. Surgery in Disorders of Sex Development (DSD) with a Gender Issue: If (Why), When and How?'" (letter). *Journal of Pediatric Urology* 12, no. 6 (2016): 438.

Mouriquand, Pierre D. E., Anthony C. Caldamone, P. Malone, J. D. Frank, and P. Hoebeke. "The ESPU/SPU Standpoint on the Surgical Management of Disorders of Sex Development (DSD)." *Journal of Pediatric Urology* 10, no. 1 (2014): 8–10.

Mouriquand, Pierre D. E., Daniela Brindusa Gorduza, Claire-Lise Gay, Heino F. L. Meyer-Bahlburg, Linda Baker, Laurence S. Baskin, et al. "Surgery in Disorders of Sex Development (DSD) with a Gender Issue: If (Why), When, and How?" *Journal of Pediatric Urology* 12, no. 3 (2016): 139–49.

Munt, Sally R. "Shame/Pride Dichotomies in *Queer as Folk*." *Textual Practice* 14, no. 3 (2000): 531–46.

Murray, Samantha. "Within or Beyond the Binary/Boundary? Intersex Infants and Parental Decisions." *Australian Feminist Studies* 24, no. 60 (2009): 265–74.

Nelson, Katherine. "The Psychological and Social Origins of Autobiographical Memory." *Psychological Science* 4, no. 1 (1993): 7–14.

Nevada, Eli, and Cheryl Chase. "Natural Allies." *Hermaphrodites with Attitude*, Summer 1995.

New, Maria. "Description and Defense of Prenatal Diagnosis and Treatment with Low-Dose Dexamethasone for Congenital Adrenal Hyperplasia." *American Journal of Bioethics* 10, no. 9 (2010): 48–51.

Newton, Esther. *Mother Camp: Female Impersonators in America*. University of Chicago Press, 1979.

Nihoul-Fékété, Claire. "Does Surgical Genitoplasty Affect Gender Identity in the Intersex Infant?" *Hormone Research* 64, supp. 2 (2005): 23–26.

Nihoul-Fékété, Claire. "How to Deal with Congenital Disorders of Sex Development in 2008 (DSD)." *European Journal of Pediatric Surgery* 18, no. 6 (2008): 364–67.

Organisation Intersex International. "Alice Dreger: Disorders of Sex Development." 2007. https://web.archive.org/web/20111216120824/http://www.intersexualite.org/AliceDreger.html.

Orr, Celeste E. "Covid and Intersex: In/Essential Medical Management." In *Covid and . . . : How to Do Rhetoric in a Pandemic*, edited by Emily Winderman, Allison L. Rowland, and Jennifer Malkowski. Michigan State University Press, 2023.

Orr, Celeste E. *Cripping Intersex*. UBC Press, 2022.

Özbey, Hüseyin, and Seref Etker. "Disorders of Sexual Development in a Cultural Context." *Arab Journal of Urology* 11, no. 1 (2013): 33–39.

Pagonis, Pidgeon. "The Son They Never Had." *Narrative Inquiry in Bioethics* 5, no. 2 (2015): 103–6.

Papageorgiou, Theocharis, Rhonda Hearns-Stokes, Dennis Peppas, and James H. Segars. "Clitoroplasty with Preservation of Neurovascular Pedicles." *Obstetrics and Gynecology* 96, no. 5 (2000): 821–23.

Parikh, Firuza Rajesh, Arundhati Sitaram Athalye, Nandkishor Jagannath Naik, Dattatray Jayaram Naik, Rupesh Ramesh Sanap, and Prochi Fali Madon. "Preimplantation Genetic Testing: Its Evolution, Where Are We Today?" *Journal of Human Reproductive Sciences* 11, no. 4 (2018): 306–14.

Park, Sungchan, Seong Heon Ha, and Kun Suk Kim. "Long-Term Follow-up After Feminizing Genital Reconstruction in Patients with Ambiguous Genitalia and High Vaginal Confluence." *Journal of Korean Medical Science* 26, no. 3 (2011): 399–403.

Pasterski, Vickie, Kiki Mastroyannopoulou, Deborah Wright, Kenneth J. Zucker, and Ieuan A. Hughes. "Predictors of Posttraumatic Stress in

Parents of Children Diagnosed with a Disorder of Sex Development." *Archives of Sexual Behavior* 43, no. 2 (2014): 369–75.

Pasterski, Vickie, Philippa Prentice, and Ieuan A. Hughes. "Consequences of the Chicago Consensus on Disorders of Sex Development (DSD): Current Practices in Europe." *Archives of Disease in Childhood* 95, no. 8 (2010): 618–23.

Pedwell, Carolyn. "Theorizing 'African' Female Genital Cutting and 'Western' Body Modifications: A Critique of the Continuum and Analogue Approaches." *Feminist Review* 86, no. 1 (2007): 45–66.

Peterson, Carole. "Children's Long-Term Memory for Autobiographical Events." *Developmental Review* 22, no. 3 (2002): 370–402.

Pitts-Taylor, Victoria. *The Brain's Body: Neuroscience and Corporeal Politics.* Duke University Press, 2016.

Preves, Sharon E. *Intersex and Identity: The Contested Self.* Rutgers University Press, 2003.

Preves, Sharon E. "Intersex Narratives: Gender, Medicine, and Identity." In *Sex, Gender, and Sexuality: The New Basics*, edited by Abby L. Ferber, Kimberly Holcomb, and Tre Wentling. Oxford University Press, 2009.

Ramachandran, V. S., and William Hirstein. "The Perception of Phantom Limbs." *Brain* 121, no. 9 (1998): 1603–30.

Rashkin, Esther. *Family Secrets and the Psychoanalysis of Narrative.* Princeton University Press, 1992.

Rashkin, Esther. *Unspeakable Secrets and the Psychoanalysis of Culture.* State University of New York Press, 2008.

Ratcliffe, Matthew. *Feelings of Being: Phenomenology, Psychiatry, and the Sense of Reality.* Oxford University Press, 2008.

Reilly, Elizabeth. "Radical Tweak—Relocating the Power to Assign Sex." *Cardozo Journal of Law and Gender* 12, no. 1 (2005): 297–336.

Reiner, William G. "Assignment of Sex in Neonates with Ambiguous Genitalia." *Current Opinion in Pediatrics* 11, no. 4 (1999): 363–65.

Reiner, William G. "To Be Male or Female—That Is the Question." *Archives of Pediatrics and Adolescent Medicine* 151, no. 3 (1997): 224–25.

Reis, Elizabeth. *Bodies in Doubt: An American History of Intersex.* 2nd ed. Johns Hopkins University Press, 2021.

Reis, Elizabeth. "Divergence or Disorder? The Politics of Naming Intersex." *Perspectives in Biology and Medicine* 50, no. 4 (2007): 535–43.

Repo, Jemima, *The Biopolitics of Gender*. Oxford University Press, 2016.

Riggs, Damien W. *Priscilla, (White) Queen of the Desert: Queer Rights/Race Privilege*. Peter Lang, 2006.

Roen, Katrina. "'But We Have to *Do Something*': Surgical 'Correction' of Atypical Genitalia." *Body & Society* 14, no. 1 (2008): 47–66.

Roen, Katrina. "Clinical Intervention and Embodied Subjectivity: Atypically Sexed Children and Their Parents." In Holmes, ed., *Critical Intersex*.

Roen, Katrina, and Vickie Pasterski. "Psychological Research and Intersex/DSD: Recent Developments and Future Directions." *Psychology and Sexuality* 5, no. 1 (2014): 102–16.

Rossiter, Katherine, and Shonna Diehl. "Gender Reassignment in Children: Ethical Conflicts in Surrogate Decision Making." *Pediatric Nursing* 24, no. 1 (1998): 59–62.

Rubin, David A. "Anger, Aggression, Attitude: Intersex Rage as Biopolitical Protest." *Signs* 46, no. 4 (2021): 987–1011.

Rubin, David A. *Intersex Matters: Biomedical Embodiment, Gender Regulation, and Transnational Activism*. State University of New York Press, 2017.

Salamon, Gayle. "Boys of the Lex: Transgenderism and Rhetorics of Materiality." *GLQ* 12, no. 4 (2006): 575–97.

Sanders, Caroline, Bernie Carter, and Lynne Goodacre. "Parents' Narratives About Their Experiences of Their Child's Reconstructive Genital Surgeries for Ambiguous Genitalia." *Journal of Clinical Nursing* 17, no. 23 (2007): 3187–95.

Sanders, Caroline, Bernie Carter, and Lynne Goodacre. "Searching for Harmony: Parents' Narratives About Their Child's Genital Ambiguity and Reconstructive Genital Surgeries in Childhood." *Journal of Advanced Nursing* 67, no. 10 (2011): 2220–30.

Scarry, Elaine. *The Body in Pain: The Making and Unmaking of the World*. Oxford University Press, 1985.

Schober, Justine Marut. "Feminization (Surgical Aspects)" (1998). In *Pediatric Surgery and Urology: Long-Term Outcomes*, 2nd ed., edited by Mark Stringer, Keith T. Oldham, and Pierre D. E. Mouriquand. Cambridge University Press, 2006.

Schober, Justine Marut. "A Surgeon's Response to the Intersex Controversy." In Dreger, ed., *Intersex in the Age of Ethics*.

Schweizer, Katinka, Franziska Brunner, Benjamin Gedrose, Christina Handford, and Hertha Richter-Appelt. "Coping with Diverse Sex

Development: Treatment Experiences and Psychosocial Support During Childhood and Adolescence and Adult Well-Being." *Journal of Pediatric Psychology* 42, no. 5 (2017): 504–19.

Seltzer, Mark. *Serial Killers: Death and Life in America's Wound Culture*. Routledge, 1998.

Shi, Tong, Yan-Kun Lin, Qiao Bao, Wei-Hua Lao, and Ke-Yu Ouyang. "One-Stage Tubularized Urethroplasty Using the Free Inner Plate of the Foreskin in the Treatment of Proximal Hypospadias." *BMC Pediatrics* 22 (2022): art. 393. https://doi.org/10.1186/s12887-022-03464-2.

Shildrick, Margrit. *Embodying the Monster: Encounters with the Vulnerable Self*. Sage, 2002.

Shildrick, Margrit. *Leaky Bodies and Boundaries: Feminism, Postmodernism, and (Bio)Ethics*. Routledge, 1997.

Shildrick, Margrit. "Unreformed Bodies: Normative Anxiety and the Denial of Pleasure." *Women's Studies* 34, nos. 3–4 (2005): 327–44.

Simmonds, Margaret. "Patients and Parents in Decision Making and Management." In *Paediatric and Adolescent Gynaecology: A Multidisciplinary Approach*, edited by Adam H. Balen, Sarah M. Creighton, Melanie C. Davies, Jane MacDougall, and Richard Stanhope. Cambridge University Press, 2004.

Simmonds, Margaret. "Was 'Variations of Reproductive Development' Considered?" (letter). *Archives of Disease in Childhood*, August 17, 2006. https://web.archive.org/web/20150514044052/http://adc.bmj.com/content/91/7/554/reply.

Slijper, Froukje M. E., Stenvert L. S. Drop, Jan C. Molenaar, and Sabine M. P. F. de Muinck Keizer-Schrama, "Long-Term Psychological Evaluation of Intersex Children." *Archives of Sexual Behavior* 27, no. 2 (1998): 125–44.

Smith, Matthew. "Where in the World Are Men Most Likely to Sit Down to Wee?" YouGov UK, May 16, 2023. https://yougov.co.uk/society/articles/45713-where-world-are-men-most-likely-sit-down-wee.

Snow, Tony. "Straight Sex Cannot Give You AIDS—Official." *Sun* (UK), November 17, 1989.

Sparrow, Robert. "Gender Eugenics? The Ethics of PGD for Intersex Conditions." *American Journal of Bioethics* 13, no. 10 (2013): 29–38.

Speiser, Phyllis W., Wiebke Arlt, Richard J. Auchus, Laurence S. Baskin, Gerard S. Conway, Deborah P. Merke, et al. "Congenital Adrenal

Hyperplasia due to Steroid 21-Hydroxylase Deficiency: An Endocrine Society Clinical Practice Guideline." *Journal of Clinical Endocrinology and Metabolism* 103, no. 11 (2018): 4043–88.

Spurgas, Alyson K. "(Un)Queering Identity: The Biosocial Production of Intersex/DSD." In Holmes, *Critical Intersex*.

Srinath, Shankarnarayan. "Identificatory Processes in Trauma." In Garland, ed., *Understanding Trauma*.

Stark, Herman E. "Authenticity and Intersexuality." In Sytsma, ed., *Ethics and Intersex*.

Stein, Martin T., David E. Sandberg, Tom Mazur, Erica Eugster, and Jorge J. Daaboul. "A Newborn Infant with a Disorder of Sexual Differentiation." *Pediatrics* 114, no. 5 (2004): 1473–77.

St-Hilaire, Colette. "Crisis and Mutation of the Apparatus of Sexuality: The Bursting of the Category of Sex" (1999). Translated by Jean Antonin Billard and Erin Mouré. *West Coast Line*, no. 35 (2001): 126–55.

Stockton, Kathryn Bond. *Beautiful Bottom, Beautiful Shame: Where "Black" Meets "Queer."* Duke University Press, 2006.

Stone, Moonhawk River. "Approaching Critical Mass: An Exploration of the Role of Intersex Allies in Creative Positive Education, Advocacy, and Change." *Cardozo Journal of Law and Gender* 12, no. 1 (2005): 352–66.

Swarr, Amanda Lock. *Envisioning African Intersex: Challenging Colonial and Racist Legacies in South African Medicine.* Duke University Press, 2023.

Sytsma, Sharon E., ed. *Ethics and Intersex.* Springer, 2006.

Tamar-Mattis, Anne. "Exceptions to the Rule: Curing the Law's Failure to Protect Intersex Infants." *Berkeley Journal of Gender, Law, and Justice* 21, no. 1 (2006): 59–110.

Tamar-Mattis, Anne. "Medical Treatment of People with Intersex Conditions as Torture and Cruel, Inhuman, or Degrading Treatment or Punishment." In *Torture in Healthcare Settings: Reflections on the Special Rapporteur on Torture's 2013 Thematic Report*, edited by Center for Human Rights and Humanitarian Law. American University, 2014.

Thomas, Barbara. "Report to AISSG on Chicago Consensus Conference October 2005." Androgen Insensitivity Syndrome Support Group, June 2006. https://web.archive.org/web/20180318023840/http://www.aissg.org/PDFs/Barbara-Chicago-Rpt.pdf.

Thrift, Nigel. *Spatial Formations.* Sage, 1996.

Timmermans, Stefan, Ashelee Yang, Melissa Gardner, Catherine E. Keegan, Beverly M. Yashar, Patricia Y. Fechner, et al. "Does Patient-Centered Care Change Genital Surgery Decisions? The Strategic Use of Clinical Uncertainty in Disorders of Sex Development Clinics." *Journal of Health and Social Behavior* 59, no. 4 (2018): 520–35.

Torok, Maria. "Story of Fear: The Symptoms of Phobia—the Return of the Repressed or the Return of the Phantom?" (1975). In Abraham and Torok, *The Shell and the Kernel.*

Truffer, Daniela. "It's a Human Rights Issue!" *Narrative Inquiry in Bioethics* 5, no. 2 (2015): 111–14.

Turton, Ailie J., and Stuart R. Butler. "Referred Sensations Following Stroke." *Neurocase* 7, no. 5 (2001): 397–405.

Vidal, Isabelle, Daniela Brindusa Gorduza, Elodie Haraux, Claire-Lise Gay, Pierre Chatelain, Marc Nicolino, et al. "Surgical Options in Disorders of Sex Development (DSD) with Ambiguous Genitalia." *Best Practice & Research Clinical Endocrinology & Metabolism* 24, no. 2 (2010): 311–24.

Vilain, Eric, John C. Achermann, Erica A. Eugster, Vincent R. Harley, Yves Morel, Jean D. Wilson, et al. "We Used to Call Them Hermaphrodites." *Genetics in Medicine* 9, no. 2 (2007): 65–66.

Viloria, Hida. *Born Both: An Intersex Life.* Hachette, 2017.

Viloria, Hida. "Promoting Health and Social Progress by Accepting and Depathologizing Benign Intersex Traits." *Narrative Inquiry in Bioethics* 5, no. 2 (2015): 114–17.

Vogler, Candace. "Much of Madness and More of Sin: Compassion, for Ligeia." In Berlant, ed., *Compassion.*

Wall, Sean Saifa. "Standing at the Intersections: Navigating Life as a Black Intersex Man." *Narrative Inquiry in Bioethics* 5, no. 2 (2015): 117–19.

Wall, Sean Saifa, and Pidgeon Pagonis. "Creating Intersex Justice: Interview with Sean Saifa Wall and Pidgeon Pagonis of the Intersex Justice Project." Interview by David A. Rubin, Michelle Wolff, and Amanda Lock Swarr. *Transgender Studies Quarterly* 9, no. 2 (2022): 187–95.

Wallin, David J. *Attachment in Psychotherapy.* Guilford, 2007.

Wang, Thelma. "Trans as Brain Intersex: The Trans–Intersex Nexus in Neurobiological Research." *Transgender Studies Quarterly* 9, no. 2 (2022): 172–83.

Warne, Garry, Sonia Grover, John Hutson, Andrew Sinclair, Sylvia Metcalfe, Elisabeth Northam, and others in the Murdoch Children's

Research Institute Sex Study Group. "A Long-Term Outcome Study of Intersex Conditions." *Journal of Pediatric Endocrinology and Metabolism* 18, no. 6 (2005): 555–67.

Warner, Michael. *The Trouble with Normal: Sex, Politics, and the Ethics of Queer Life.* Harvard University Press, 1999.

Wartenberg, Thomas E. *The Forms of Power: From Domination to Transformation.* Temple University Press, 1990.

Weber, Daniel M., Verena B. Schönbucher, Markus A. Landolt, and Rita Gobet. "The Pediatric Penile Perception Score: An Instrument for Patient Self-Assessment and Surgeon Evaluation After Hypospadias Repair." *Journal of Urology* 180, no. 3 (2008): 1080–84.

Wee, Amanda, Tapasi Bagchi, and Rebecca Kimble. "Creation and Maintenance of Neo-Vagina with the Use of Vaginal Dilators as First Line Treatment: Results from a Quaternary Paediatric and Adolescent Gynaecology Service in Australia." *Australian and New Zealand Journal of Obstetrics and Gynaecology* 62, no. 3 (2022): 439–44.

Weiss, Meira. "Fence Sitters: Parents' Reactions to Sexual Ambiguities in Their Newborn Children." *Semiotica* 107, nos. 1–2 (1995): 33–50.

Werner, Ralf, Helga Grötsch, and Olaf Hiort. "46,XY Disorders of Sex Development—the Undermasculinised Male with Disorders of Androgen Action." *Best Practice & Research Clinical Endocrinology & Metabolism* 24, no. 2 (2010): 263–77.

Whittle, Stephen. "Gender Fucking or Fucking Gender?" (1996). In Morland and Willox, eds., *Queer Theory.*

Wiesemann, Claudia, Susanne Ude-Koeller, Gernot H. G. Sinnecker, and Ute Thyen. "Ethical Principles and Recommendations for the Medical Management of Differences of Sex Development (DSD)/Intersex in Children and Adolescents." *European Journal of Pediatrics* 169, no. 6 (2010): 671–79.

Wilcox, D. T., and P. G. Ransley. "Medicolegal Aspects of Hypospadias." *BJU International* 86, no. 3 (2000): 327–31.

Wingrove, Elizabeth. "Interpellating Sex." *Signs* 24, no. 4 (1999): 869–93.

Wolff, Michele, David A. Rubin, and Amanda Lock Swarr. "The Intersex Issue: An Introduction." *Transgender Studies Quarterly* 9, no. 2 (2022): 143–59.

Wolffenbuttel, K. P., and Naomi S. Crouch. "Timing of Feminising Surgery in Disorders of Sex Development." In *Understanding Differences and*

Disorders of Sex Development (DSD), edited by Olaf Hiort and S. Faisal Ahmed. Karger, 2014.

Young, Iris Marion. "The Scaling of Bodies and the Politics of Identity" (1990). In *Space, Gender, Knowledge: Feminist Readings*, edited by Linda McDowell and Joanne P. Sharp. Arnold, 1997.

Young, Iris Marion. "Throwing Like a Girl: A Phenomenology of Feminine Body Comportment, Motility, and Spatiality" (1980). In *Throwing Like a Girl and Other Essays in Feminist Philosophy and Social Theory*. Indiana University Press, 1990.

Zeiler, Kristin, and Anette Wickström. "Why Do 'We' Perform Surgery on Newborn Intersexed Children? The Phenomenology of the Parental Experience of Having a Child with Intersex Anatomies." *Feminist Theory* 10, no. 3 (2009): 359–77.

Ziemińska, Renata. "Toward a Nonbinary Model of Gender/Sex Traits." *Hypatia* 37, no. 2 (2022): 402–21.

Zieselman, Kimberly M. *XOXY: A Memoir*. Jessica Kingsley, 2020.

Zilberstein, Karen. "Neurocognitive Considerations in the Treatment of Attachment and Complex Trauma in Children." *Clinical Child Psychology and Psychiatry* 19, no. 3 (2014): 336–54.

Zucker, Kenneth J., Susan J. Bradley, Gillian Oliver, Jennifer Blake, Susan Fleming, and Jane Hood. "Self-Reported Sexual Arousability in Women with Congenital Adrenal Hyperplasia." *Journal of Sex and Marital Therapy* 30, no. 5 (2004): 343–55.

INDEX

Fixing Sex (Karkazis), 19

Foster, Hal, 70

Foucault, Michel: on power and
knowledge, 112, 148, 150; on
sexual politics, 230n17

Fraser, Nancy, 240n77

Freeman, Elizabeth, 112, 122–23; on
temporal drag, 128

Freud, Sigmund, 101, 225n39; on
repression, 98

Fuckology (Downing, Morland, and
Sullivan), 6

gender, 14; determinants of,
22–23, 28, 52, 56; as defensive
identification, 91; in feminism,
108, 110; in medicine, 2, 4, 21,
48, 58–59, 85, 132, 177;
performativity, 127, 182; in
queer theory, 110–11; as
trauma, 69, 71

Gender Trouble (Butler), 182

genitals: clitoris, 1, 3, 4, 106, 127,
140, 142, 197; gonads, 1, 166–69,
226n42; penis, 1, 4, 19, 127, 132,
139, 143; postsurgical, 26, 72, 114,
127, 147–48, 191; as protected
characteristics, 211n31; in
psychoanalysis, 92–93; vagina,
52, 141

Germany, 198

Germon, Jenz, 140

Gill-Peterson, Jules, 235n22

Grabham, Emily, 22, 238n50

Grace, Victoria, 189

Greece, 198

Griffiths, David Andrew, 233n68

Groveman, Sherri A., 140

Grumbach, Melvin, 188, 193, 247n71

Halberstam, Jack, 118–19, 129–30

Halley, Janet E., 212n33

Halperin, David M., 115, 122; on
Foucault, 112–13, 229–30n17

Hermaphrodites with Attitude
(Intersex Society of North
America), 53

hermaphroditism, terminology of,
166–67

Hermer, Laura D., 213n40

Herndon, April M., 172

Hird, Myra J., 140

history, 122, 131–34

History of Sexuality, The (Foucault),
112

Hollibaugh, Amber, 131

Holmes, M. Morgan, 21, 167; on
medical power, 141; on medical
terminology, 186; on patient
narratives, 51; on surgery, 128,
191; on trauma, 73

homophobia, 50, 115

Horkheimer, Max, 239n64

hormones, 1, 52, 143, 176;
dexamethasone, 74, 240n73;
testosterone, 197

Houk, Christopher P., 190–92

human rights, 4–5, 29, 183, 234n10

Iceland, 198

identity: and diagnosis, 32, 173–75;
intersex as, 5, 53, 119, 176;
politics, 26–27. See also gender

ideology, 157–58

GPSR Authorized Representative: Easy Access System Europe, Mustamäe tee 50, 10621 Tallinn, Estonia, gpsr.requests@easproject.com